THE
MEDICAL
RUNAROUND

THE
MEDICAL
RUNAROUND

DR. ANDREW MALLESON

HART PUBLISHING COMPANY, INC.
NEW YORK CITY

CONTENTS

You have been deceived.
They have made promises
    and failed to fulfill them.
You want dignity; they give
    you money.
You want a future with hope—
    they give you despair.
You must fight for a future
    with dignity.

A POSTER ON A WALL

I do my thing, and you do your thing.
I am not in this world to live up to your expectations.
And you are not in this world to live up to mine.
You are you, and I am I;
And if by chance we find each other, it's beautiful.
If not, it can't be helped.

FREDERICK S. PERLS

ACKNOWLEDGMENTS

The author wishes to thank the following publishers for permission to use copyrighted material from their books:

Philosophical Library: A. A. Roback and Thomas Kierman, *The Pictorial History of Psychology and Psychiatry*, New York, 1969.

International Scientific Press: H. J. Eysenck, *The Effects of Psychotherapy*, New York, 1966.

J. and A. Churchill: Dr. D. R. Laurence, *Clinical Pharmacology*, London, 1966.

Williams and Wilkins: James H. Huddleson, *Accidents, Neurosis and Compensation*, Baltimore, 1932.

Faber and Faber: T. S. Eliot, *The Four Quartets*, London, 1944.

John Wright and Son: Russel Barton, *Institutional Neurosis*, Bristol, 1959.

Bell Publishing Co.: Thomas Szasz, *The Myth of Mental Illness*, New York, 1961.

Lyle Stuart: Ferdinand Lundberg, *The Rich and the Super Rich*, New York, 1968.

Real People Press: Frederick S. Perls, *Gestalt Therapy Verbatim*, California, 1969.

Ferdinand Enke: Eugen Höllander, *Die Karikatur und Satire in der Medizin*, Stuttgart, 1905.

The author also wishes to thank Dr. J. Womersley, Dr. Nathan Klein, Dr. Moya Woodside, and Dr. H. Bourne for permission to use their letters to medical journals.

The author wishes to thank the editors of and authors published in the following journals and periodicals for permission to use their material:

Proceedings of the Royal Society of Medicine: Neil Kessel and W. McCullock, "Repeated Acts of Self-Poisoning and Self-Injury," *59,* 89 (1966).

Globe and Mail of Canada: Farrell Crook, "Mental Patients Denied Meals," Toronto, June 17, 1970.

Bulletin of Narcotics: Thomas Bewley, "Estimate of the Incidence of Drug Abuse in the United Kingdom," *13,* 1967.

Playboy Magazine: Lenny Bruce, "How to Talk Dirty and Influence People," November 1963.

Archives of General Psychiatry: Arnold M. Ludwig and Frank Farrelly, "The Code of Chronicity," *15,* 562 (1966).

The Scientific American: Christopher Tietze and Sarah Lewit, "Abortion," *220* (1), 21 (1969).

Journal of Psychosomatic Research: Neil Kessel, "The Respectability of Self-Poisoning and the Fashion for Survival," *10,* 29 (1966).

British Medical Journal: Neil Kessel, "Self-Poisoning," *4,* 1268 (1965).

The author would like to thank Dr. Frances Frank, Dr. Norman Angel, Dr. Nick Barnes, Dr. Henry Durost, and Mrs. Kit Stewart for reading his manuscript, clarifying some of his ideas, improving his grammar, and correcting his spelling:

Most of all, the author would like to thank Mrs. Amy Ruth, the librarian of the Queen Street Mental Health Centre, for her kind and patient help, and for her remarkable ability to ferret out all sorts of information.

A list of all individuals, companies, and institutions to whom I am indebted for illustrations will be found at the end of the book.

INTRODUCTION

We all want a society of sane, free, and healthy people. Doctors deal with diseases; sometimes competently, but often not. Today's medical profession is the child of the early barber-surgeons and the quack magicians whose traditions die hard.

Sociologists, biologists, psychologists, and many other professionals are also interested in disease and in health. All these professionals influence our ideas about illness and influence the ways in which we are treated when we are sick.

Health issues are vote-catching, and politicians argue and legislate about matters of health. Ill health is big business. Doctors and many others make their living because of ill health, and pharmaceutical firms make fortunes.

All Western countries are now engaged in exciting experiments in health care. How well are these working? Can these proposals be improved?

Hippocrates, the great father of medicine, taught above all things that doctors should be useful to their patients, and should do their clients no harm. Medical care is expensive; it certainly affects our pockets, if not our persons. Does the money we spend today on medical care buy us a useful service? How useful are doctors and their medicines? Could doctors be *more* useful? These questions are the subject of this book.

A Doctor at Work

A young man visits his doctor complaining of abdominal pain. The doctor examines him and finds the right side of the abdomen tender. He sends him to a hospital. The young man has an inflamed appendix removed. Several days later, having recovered, he is discharged. He has been saved from an illness which, had it not been treated, would probably have been fatal. He and society have received a useful service. No one would object save those who believe in no human intervention.

But comparatively few patients seen in general practice come to the doctor with such a life-threatening illness. The common cold is the illness that the general practitioner most commonly sees. Many of his patients do not have a physical illness at all, but a psychiatric one.

What is meant by a psychiatric illness? Let us look at some young men whose appendixes and other organs are normal, but who nevertheless complain of abdominal pain.

After a sexual adventure, one young man thinks he has VD. Not knowing what symptoms to expect, to him every abdominal gurgle portends disaster. Discomfort is nurtured into pain. Not daring to confess the cause of his concern, he vaguely hopes that the doctor will, by looking at him, be able to refute his fears.

Another young man is dangled on a string by his girlfriend. His anxiety runs high. This gives him abdominal pain, and he complains to his doctor.

A third believes that a snake lives in his abdomen. He does not like the pain that this causes.

15

A fourth wants to go to a football match; a doctor's certificate will help fix things up with his employer.

A fifth hopes to be given sleeping pills.

A sixth belongs to a small but well-recognized group of young men who just like having operations. His abdomen is already crisscrossed by numerous scars—a hallmark of his love-affair with surgery.

A seventh fractured his skull in a car accident years ago. The scarring in his brain causes an unusual form of epileptic attack which starts with abdominal discomfort and goes on to produce a transient feeling of apprehension. The feeling is unpleasant, and since the attack is always preceded by abdominal pain, the sufferer believes the pain to be the cause of the epilepsy and complains of the pain to his doctor.

The last young man just bellyaches.

All these young men have a disorder of either brain, mind, or behavior. Traditionally—but quite arbitrarily—all these complaints are labeled psychiatric. Minor physical illnesses, such as the cold, and psychiatric disorders constitute the bulk of a general practitioner's work. Oddly enough, *most general practitioners have not been trained in the management of either of these two conditions.*

Doctors in the Making

General medical training is much the same all over the world. The course takes about six years. During the first half of his training, the medical student learns basic sciences: chemistry, physics, biology, physiology, and biochemistry. For 18 months or so, he learns anatomy and he smells of corpses. In the second half of his training, he learns clinical practice from specialists who teach on patients ill enough to be in a hospital.

Teaching hospitals are concerned with the diagnosis and treatment of serious physical disease. Such institutions cater particularly to patients with unusual disorders. So while the student may become familiar with the treatment of tsutsuga-mushi fever, he is unlikely to see, except by accident, a patient with a common cold.

Neither does the student-doctor learn much psychiatry. Patients in teaching hospitals certainly have their fair share of psychiatric problems, but the staff is seldom concerned with those matters. Interest centers on the number of operations that a man has had, not in the number of his wives. The student gets little opportunity to learn about the common problems of family conflicts, let alone learn what—if anything—should be done about them.

Most patients want their colds and their other minor illnesses treated. They want advice on how to deal with a nagging wife or a rebellious child. But, there is no reason why a newly turned out doctor should be any better at curing colds or dealing with a nagging wife than anybody else. He certainly has not learned anything about the management of minor physical disorders, nor has he learned how to deal with embattled families and with human unhappiness.

He soon learns from his patients.

Pills and Sympathy

"Doctor, I've got a cold again. I need some of those drops for my nose—the ones that smart. Some of those green and pink pills that my neighbor has to dry up her running nose. I ought to have some phenacetins for the muscle ache. And, Doctor, I need some of that syrup for the cough—it's red. Oh, you'll find the name on my card—the other doctor gave me some for my last cold."

The new doctor also learns what pills to give to the miserable among his patients, and how to tell his patients to be happy.

Do his treatments work?

And how useful is his psychiatry?

Most of his treatments probably do not work, and most of his psychiatry is probably pretty useless.

SOURCES

Bynoe, M. L.: "The Common Cold." *Practitioner*, **197** 739 (1966).

Goldberg, D. P., and Blackwell, B.: "Psychiatric Illness in General Practice." *British Medical Journal*, **2** 439 (1970).

Fashions in Treatment

People have always been determined to get medical treatment. And sometimes downright odd about what they want and what they are willing to accept. Flip through old textbooks of therapeutics in some second-hand bookshop, or just look at the illustrations in this volume. The purge, the cautery, and the enema syringe must have hurried many of our ancestors to a painful and unnecessarily early end, but the survivors were not deterred. They insisted on being purged and cauterized to the end.

Hippocrates wrote:

Those diseases which medicines do not cure are cured by the knife; those diseases that the knife does not cure are cured by the cautery; and those diseases that the cautery does not cure are incurable.

The cautery and the seton were used on the principle that pain or disease of the body could be cured by providing a further discomfort—"a counter irritation." The cautery was a branding iron, and the seton was a bristle or strand of horse hair which was threaded through the skin and left to fester for several months.

The cautery and the seton remained trusted treatments for 3,000 years or so. The popularity of the cautery waned toward the end of the 18th century, and the seton stopped being used about a hundred years ago.

Treatments keep up with science, and new scientific discoveries are soon incorporated into the treatment mystique. In the 1860s Lord Joseph Lister revolutionalized surgery with his discovery that carbolic acid kills bacteria. Surgery became aseptic and much safer. The "Carbolic Smoke Ball" soon burst upon the public. Its manufacturers claimed that it would positively cure: colds, catarrh, asthma, bronchitis, hoarseness, loss of voice, influenza, hay fever, throat deafness, sore throat, snoring, croup, whooping cough, neuralgia, and headache. Support for their claims was given by three English marchionesses, twelve countesses and many other lesser members of the English aristocracy. But of the diseases its manufacturers claimed that the smoke ball could cure, not many were even caused by bacteria, and in any event the inhalation of its fumes could not possibly have killed the offending bacteria.

When at the end of the last century electricity was still a novelty, cures became "electric." Magnets were placed in suspensory belts, hair brushes and garters—the term electric was even added to pills and medicines to make them sparkle. There were virtually no diseases left that these electric treatments were not claimed to cure.

The Enema

Most fashions start at the top of society, and medical treatment is no exception. Fashionable 17th-century France was a trend setter. In one year, Louis XIII had 212 enemas, 215 purgations, and 47 bleedings. With Louis XIV, the enema came into its own. It became a household ritual; most upper-class people had one every day. A celebrated legal case concerned payment for the administration of 2,190 enemas within two years to a canon of Troyes.

The fashion spread to England and America. The more frugal, using an assortment of devices, administered their own.

Constipation

Our Victorian great-grandparents were preoccupied with their

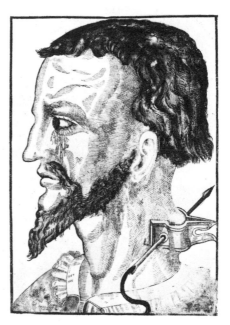

This 16th century drawing shows the use of the seton to cure a running eye.

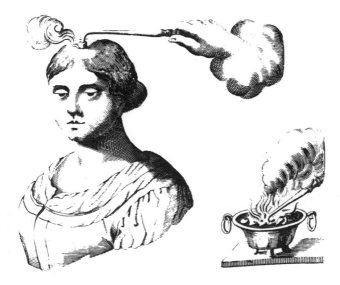

The cautery is being used to cure a headache. When so used its application had to be gentle so as not to risk roasting the brain or shriveling up its membranes.

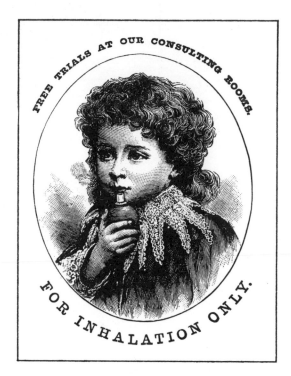

Lister discovered that carbolic acid kills germs, and the "Carbolic Smoke Ball" burst upon the public. Most skin diseases are not caused by germs. Carbolic is a skin irritant, and this carbolic salve must have made many skin diseases worse.

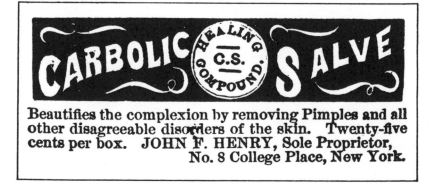

bowels. Constipation was treated with every conceivable concoction. By the early years of the 20th century, Sir Arbuthnot Lane had perfected an operation for removal of the large intestine as a cure for constipation. The miseries of constipated colons were replaced by those of continual diarrhea. Sir Arbuthnot himself performed over a thousand of these operations.

Tonsillectomy

Fashion in treatment concentrated next on tonsils. Doctors cut them out wholesale. Ear, nose, and throat surgeons became the richest of all specialists, as the operation proved a popular treatment for children. American parents were as enthusiastic about tonsillectomy as the British, who by 1930, were slicing out the tonsils of nearly three-quarters of their children.

It is normal for children to have large tonsils. Tonsils grow smaller with age. Which children—if any—should have tonsillectomies?

The American Child Health Association demonstrated that a constant percentage of all children are regarded as suitable candidates. Of a thousand 11-year-old children surveyed in the New York City public school system, 61 percent had had their tonsils removed. The 390 who still had their tonsils were then referred to physicians, who recommended tonsillectomy for 45 percent of these 390 children. The remainder were then referred to another group of physicians who selected 46 percent of these children for tonsillectomy. The rejected 54 percent were, in their turn, sent to yet another group of physicians, who then selected 44 percent of those remaining. After three examinations, only 65 children out of 390 (actually 65 out of 1,000) had not been recommended for tonsillectomy. The experiment was not continued—no other school physicians were left to examine the remaining 65 children.

Careful follow-up studies have shown that only in special circumstances is a child's health improved by a tonsillectomy. For the great majority of children, this "routine" operation has no beneficial effects. It does not even diminish the incidence of common colds.

Tonsils are a part of the body's defense system against dis-

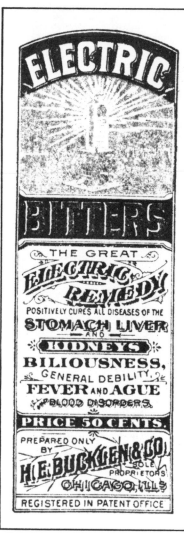
When electricity began to brighten our lives it also made our treatments sparkle.

ease; so, not surprisingly, those children who have had their tonsils removed are more vulnerable to infection. A fourfold increase in the incidence of bulbar polio, the most lethal form of poliomyelitis, has been reported among persons who had had their tonsils out compared to those who have not undergone this operation.

A 1971 study showed that people who have undergone tonsillectomies are 2.9 times more likely to develop Hodgkin's disease, a fatal cancerous condition of young adults.

Tonsillectomy is a frightening operation. Not only do children who have been subjected to it develop all sorts of psychological disturbances, but the operation is a particularly dangerous one. Postoperative bleeding can be heavy, and may go unnoticed until it is too late. In 1962, the British Ministry of Health reported 13 deaths in 18,356 operations. In the United States, the mortality rate is even higher: for every thousand children who have their tonsils out, one child dies. An additional 16 are made seriously ill.

A 1970 estimate predicts five deaths each year for every 800,000 women who use "the Pill." In other words, it is as dangerous for an American child to have his tonsils out as it is for his mother to be on the Pill for 160 years.

Or, since the death rate from abortion in New York City hospitals is eight deaths per 100,000 operations, it is 12 times more dangerous for a New York child to have his tonsils out than it is for his mother to have an abortion.

Despite this, a mother who is far too anxious about the dangers of the Pill to take it, or who would not dream of submitting herself to the dangers of an abortion, will distrust doctors who are reluctant to take out her child's tonsils. But the Pill and abortion, of course, are *preventive* measures. Tonsillectomy is *treatment*, and that makes it special.

Pharmacopoeia

Medicine was once based mostly upon magic. Much of it still is. Plato believed that the womb or "hysteros" ardently de-

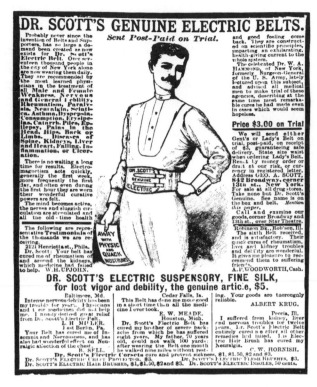

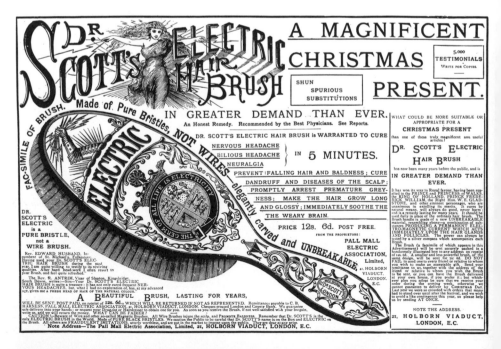

sired to produce children. If a woman remained sterile for long after puberty, her womb became indignant, dissatisfied, and even ill-tempered, and would wander through her body causing mischief or hysteria. For the treatment of hysteria, Hippocrates recommended valerian, which being the most horrible-tasting medicine known to man, was guaranteed to drive the womb back to its rightful place. In England, some doctors still use a mixture of valerian and bromide as a treatment for the miseries of menopause.

In the 16th century, men believed in the doctrine of "signatures," that is that the appearance of plants revealed their healing qualities. The quivering aspen was given for the shaking palsy because its leaves trembled. Plants with cordate leaves were good for heart disease, thistles were prescribed for a stitch in the side, and walnut shells for head injuries.

The long-preserved flesh of ancient Egyptian mummies was once considered a sure way of preserving life, and in 17th-century Europe, a brisk trade was conducted in "medical mummies." During epidemics, supplies from Alexandria ran short,

Health without physic, and the angels sing.

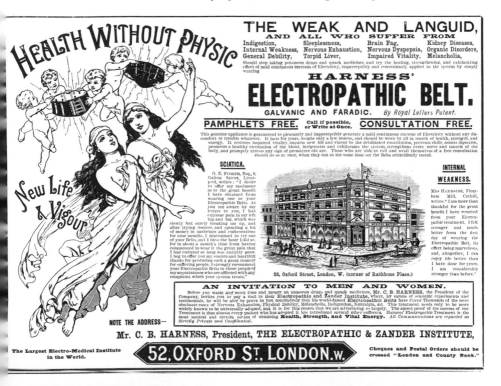

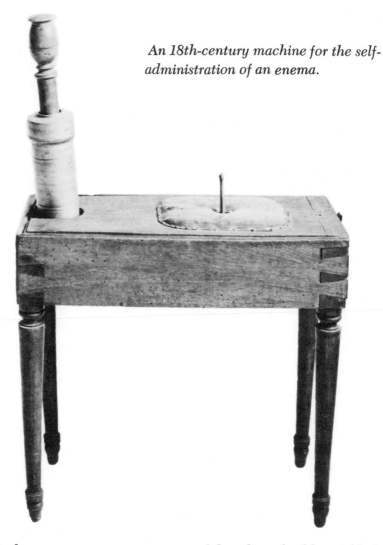

An 18th-century machine for the self-administration of an enema.

and there were some nasty scandals when freshly pickled slaves were substituted. So began our pharmacopoeia.

Magic and antiquated attitudes are still too typical of medicine. Drugs such as penicillin are scientific marvels, but their use in many instances is less than scientific.

A doctor sees a child with a streptococcal sore throat. He prescribes penicillin, which is very good at killing streptococci, and the child quickly recovers. But most sore throats are not caused by streptococci; they are caused by viruses. Viruses grow happily in the presence of penicillin; so dosing with penicillin does not help a virus sore throat to recover—the throat will do so anyway within a few days.

Nevertheless, many doctors prescribe penicillin for *all* sore throats because it is known to be a potent drug and a "good treatment." And, of course, the penicillin has accomplished something: the doctor has another grateful patient.

The New Drugs

Treatments given to satisfy patients who would feel cheated without prescribed medication are called placebos. Ethical doctors do not like prescribing biologically inert substances be-

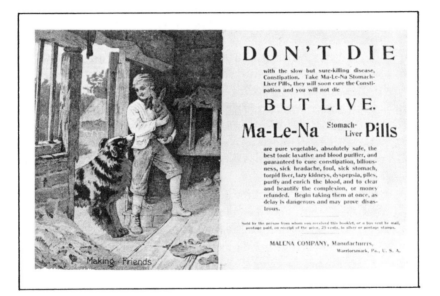

The general preoccupation with digestive and rectal ailments continued into the 19th and early 20th centuries. Ma-le-na pills were guaranteed to save you from the "sure-killing disease, Constipation." If these pills contained mercury, as many others did, the constipation did indeed become a killer.

cause this seems too much a deception. They prefer to prescribe one of the new products of the burgeoning pharmaceutical industry. These biologically potent drugs are known to at least *do* something.

This "something" may be good. But for the very reason that these drugs are biologically active, they may also do harm. A patient given an active drug for the wrong reasons will receive none of its benefits and will be exposed only to its dangers.

Iatrogenic Diseases

Diseases caused by doctors and their activities are called iatrogenic diseases. They are also known as DOMP, for *Diseases of Medical Practice*. DOMP is now common. An adverse drug reaction has been a major factor in 4 percent of all admissions to United States hospitals. And once in a hospital, a patient's chance of getting DOMP increases.

In one American teaching hospital, 20 percent of all patients contracted DOMP. In 5 percent of these cases, DOMP was serious enough to be life-threatening—if not fatal. The chances of a patient developing DOMP were directly proportional to the time of exposure to the hazard, i.e., the time he stayed in the hospital.

British doctors are considerably more conservative in the use of drugs than are American physicians. Nevertheless, a similar survey in a Belfast hospital showed that of 1,160 patients who received drugs, more than 10 percent had an adverse reaction. Sir Derrick Dunlop, a doctor and former chairman of the Committee on Drug Safety in Britain, writes that "probably 10 percent of our patients suffer to a greater or lesser extent from our efforts to treat them."

One of the lethal paradoxes of medical practice is that if a doctor decides he can do no better than nature and withholds treatments, he is likely to be regarded by the patient or by his relatives as uncaring; if the untreated patient dies, he may be regarded as criminal. If the patient dies under treatment, then

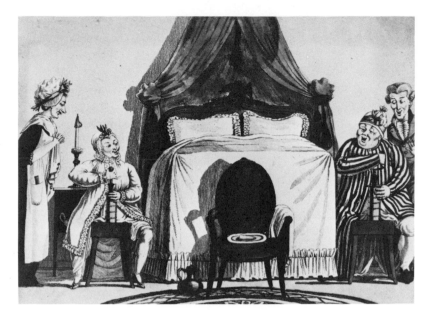

Madame and monsieur douche themselves before going to bed. During the reign of Louis XIV, an enema a day was thought to keep the doctor away.

the doctor is regarded as just unlucky. "The doctor did his best," or the disease was incurable. Doctors do not like resentful relatives, questioning coroners, and threatened litigation. They treat.

Getting Hooked

People have always been prone to getting hooked on drugs. If you could ask your great-grandmother what would happen if she stopped taking her nightly concoction of blue pill, calomel, aloes, colocynth, and her castor and croton oils, your impropriety and stupidity might get you a clip on the head. Of course, her bowels would not move for a month!

The body is a self-regulating machine. If dosed regularly with purgatives, a body just does not go on having diarrhea; it accommodates to its new circumstances, and after a few weeks, returns to its original habits. In pharmacological parlance, "tolerance" has developed.

To a Victorian, those original habits were unacceptably sluggish. The bowel had to be kept constantly in trim by repeatedly increasing the size of one's nightly dose. If an enlightened doctor—and there were some—stopped this nightly concoction of purgatives, accommodation again had to take place, this time to the absence of the drugs. Your costive relative would by fashionable injunction have been "out of sorts," would have dismissed the enlightened doctor, and would have returned to her purgatives.

Enlightened Victorian physicians certainly did complain about the harmful effects of purgatives. Dr. R. J. Graves, who first described thyrotoxicosis, also known as Graves' disease, wrote in his *Clinical Lectures:*

> *Various causes have combined to render blue pill and calomel almost popular remedies to which many have recourse when their bowels are irregular, or the stomach out of order. Indeed, it is quite incredible what a number of persons are in the habit of taking these preparations, either singularly or in combination with other preparations, whenever, to use the common expression, they find themselves bilious. The habit sooner or later induces a state of extreme nervous irritability, and the invalid finally becomes a confirmed and unhappy hypochrondriac; he is, in fact slowly poisoned without the more obvious symptoms of mercurialization being at any time produced.*

Blue pill and calomel contain mercury, which is poisonous.

In spite of a vigorous rearguard action waged by television commercials, most of us are no longer obsessed with the dangers of constipation, and the popularity of Victorian blockbusting has waned.

Calomel, one of these blockbusters, did remain in use until recently as a constituent of the teething powders with which anxious mothers treated their babies.

"Pink disease" was a serious and not uncommon disease of infants and small children. First described in 1903, this disease baffled medical science for nearly half a century. Then, in 1948, two groups of researchers independently discovered mercury in the urine of babies suffering from pink disease. The mercury poisoning was traced to the calomel in teething powders. Many countries then banned calomel from such powders, and pink disease is now very rare.

"To Medicine Thee to That Sweet Sleep"

Fashions change. Purgatives were necessary for our great-grandparents, and sleeping pills are necessary for us. It is impossible to know what percentage of Victorian bowel movements was drug induced, nor do we actually know what percentage of our sleep is drug induced. Sir Derrick Dunlop calculates that enough sleeping pills are distributed in Great Britain to induce 10 percent of all the sleep of British men, women, and *children.* And Americans are even fonder of sleeping pills than the British.

"No small art is it to sleep," said Nietzsche. Doctors help by prescribing large quantities of pills. Are all these pills useful? Evidence is accumulating that they are, in fact, just the opposite. Many who complain of poor sleep often sleep better than they think they do. Objective experiment in a sleep laboratory has shown that "bad" sleepers average only 45 minutes less sleep per night than do "good" sleepers.

Insomnia, like constipation, depends almost entirely upon an arbitrary assessment by an individual of how *he* thinks things ought to be. Many just "feel" that they do not sleep enough, and therefore believe that they need sleeping pills to make them sleep longer.

Sleeping pills do work for a while, but then they stop doing so. Just as great-grandmother developed a tolerance to purgatives, so does the "poor" sleeper develop a tolerance to sleeping pills, till they no longer lengthen the normal period of his sleep. Tolerance generally begins to develop after 10 nights of their regular use, and is complete after three months. The "poor" sleeper then has to take more pills if he wants longer sleep. Tolerance again develops to the higher dose. In this way, the user is tempted into taking ever increasing amounts of the drug.

When the size of the regular nightly dose approaches the size of the lethal dose, accidents happen. Of the 10,000 deaths from barbiturate poisoning that occur in the United States every year, it is estimated that half are accidental.

Great-grandmother became dependent upon purgatives to move a recalcitrant bowel. The regular user of hypnotics becomes dependent upon his sleeping pills for his night's sleep. When great-grandmother stopped taking her purgatives, she became terribly constipated. When the regular user of hypnotics stops taking his pills, he develops terrible insomnia. If he has used these drugs for a long time, it may take several weeks or months before his sleeping pattern returns to normal.

For 18 consecutive nights, two volunteers were given a fairly large dose of barbiturates. On stopping the drug, one, volunteer averaged only three and one half hours' sleep for the next three nights, and both suffered nightmares for the next two weeks.

Patients who are prescribed sleeping pills soon get hooked. Is there a hazard in taking sleeping pills regularly? A survey of the use of barbiturates among a general practice of 10,000 patients found that in a two-month period 407 patients were prescribed barbiturates. Of these, 58 percent had taken the pills for more than one year. The most characteristic finding among these patients was that they had developed chronic psychiatric and physical complaints that defied accepted treatment, and that they all demanded increasing dosages of barbiturates.

It is the story of the chicken and the egg. Patients who have been on barbiturates for years are miserable. Did their misery lead them to take barbiturates in the first place, or are they miserable because they take these depressant drugs? Undoubtedly, depressed and anxious people use barbiturates more frequently than do others; but there is evidence that barbiturates ultimately induce more anxiety and more depression. Some chronic users—when they allow themselves to be weaned off these drugs—do, after a few weeks, feel much better.

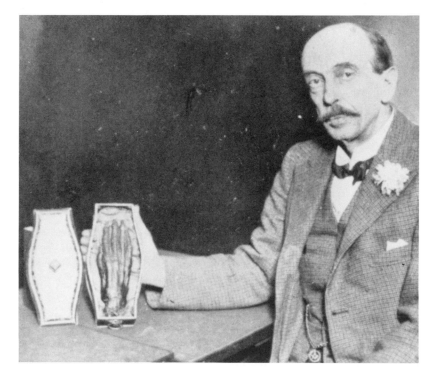

People have so much faith in their doctors that new "cures" almost invariably work; tests have demonstrated that about a third of all patients claim improvement no matter what treatment their doctor gives them. This mummified hand, for instance, is alleged to be that of an Egyptian princess of 4,000 years ago. Its owners claim that the hand has cured more than 600 sick people.

Brain Poison

Regular use of hypnotics can addle the brains of the elderly. Harry Solomon, professor of psychiatry at Harvard University, became a legend for his success in treating patients over 50 who were confused and forgetful. All he did was take them off their barbiturates. He ultimately banned all barbiturates from his hospital; and many patients who were assumed to be suffering from chronic brain disease became much more competent.

Perhaps sleeping pills also addle the brains of the future generation. Everyone knows of the tragic results of the use of thalidomide by women in the first three months of pregnancy. Doctors and drug firms now conscientiously advise that sleeping pills should not be used in the first three months of pregnancy; but animal experiments suggest that sleeping pills other than thalidomide are more likely to be harmful during the *last* three months of pregnancy. The offspring of rats treated during pregnancy with barbiturates are less able to solve feed-finding mazes than are the offspring of untreated rats. Presumably, this impairment of rat intelligence is caused by the damaging effects of barbiturates on the developing brain.

Barbiturates and other sleeping pills are, after all, brain poisons. Tissues are at their most vulnerable to the effects of poisons at a time when the tissues grow fastest. The most rapid brain growth in the rat occurs after birth; but in humans, the most rapid growth occurs during the few weeks surrounding birth. It is reasonable to assume that the developing brain in the last few weeks of human pregnancy is even more susceptible to damage by barbiturates and other sleeping medication than is the brain of the foetal rat. If the mother takes such drugs at this time, they will interfere with the development of the baby's brain and the intelligence of her child.

The U.S. Food and Drug Administration prohibited the use of thalidomide because it was suspected that thalidomide interfered with the chemistry of the thyroid gland. Some European countries were not so cautious, but four years and 10,500 deformed babies later (in West Germany and England), the association between the use of thalidomide in pregnancy and the births of limbless babies was noticed.

Hypnotics are prescribed for large numbers of women to help them cope with the sleepless nights of late pregnancy. How long will it take us to determine whether a few points have been knocked off a child's IQ because the mother took sleeping pills in late pregnancy? Only through extensive investigation will we be able to be sure that what happens in rats does not also happen in humans. Are humans so intelligent that we can afford to take that chance?

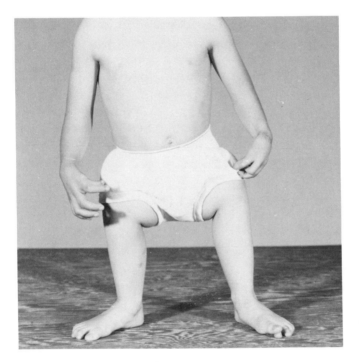

No amount of therapy will prepare this victim of thalidomide for a productive role in society. Although thalidomide is no longer on the market, other hypnotics are being prescribed for pregnant women, with untold effect on their children.

Attacking Our Friends

Most of the standard treatments prescribed in general practice for minor physical illnesses are not only contrary to the principles of scientific medicine, but are contrary to common sense. The therapeutic attack is delivered, not against the *cause* of the disease, but against the *symptoms* that the disease causes. Yet these symptoms often constitute the body's defense mechanisms against the disease-causing agent. Recovery takes place —not because of, but in spite of treatment.

Through eons of evolution, our bodies have developed defense mechanisms against the invasion of microbes and against damage by harmful chemicals. These mechanisms are wonderfully successful, for we survive many such onslaughts. Potentially dangerous mucus in the trachea is expelled by a protective cough. Noxious substances in the gut are voided by the intestinal hurry of diarrhea. Invasion of the body by germs is accompanied by a rise in body temperature. This rise in temperature probably increases the rate at which the body's chemical defense mechanisms can be mobilized. But what happens when a patient visits his doctor?

The physician treats the coughs with a cough medicine, which is either an expectorant to make the patient cough, or a cough syrup to stop the patient from doing so. An expectorant does not make us cough up phlegm any better than does a hot cup of tea, and it often makes us feel sick. Fortunately, cough syrups hardly work at all; if they did, the common cold would be a hazardous disease. We would all be in danger of drowning in our own secretions. But since these syrups are really only adulterated sugar water, all they do is fatten the already overweight and coat children's teeth with sugar.

Cough syrups were once even more syrupy, but sometime during the last century, they were thinned in St. Bartholomew's, a most prestigious London teaching hospital, after it was discovered that the local children were selling their cough syrup for a penny to an old lady who made jam tarts with it. Then other hospitals followed suit.

Today's doctor has several treatments for diarrhea, most of which are reprehensible. The standard treatment is a mixture of either chalk or clay and opium. The chalk and clay are given on the old supposition that they absorb toxins—which they do not—and the opium is given because it slows down peristaltic action—which it does. I find no discussion in the medical literature about possible harmful effects of this.

During my first day as a junior doctor in a hospital for infectious diseases, I prescribed this standard clay and opium mixture. On the second day, I was sent for by the old and crotchety but very experienced medical superintendent who called me a murderer. By abolishing the diarrhea, I was encouraging the food-poisoning bacteria to remain in the body and enter the bloodstream. I was converting an innocuous condition into one which might have been fatal.

Antibiotics and other bacteriocidal drugs are the modern favored treatments for diarrhea. Drug firms stress that these drugs can eradicate harmful bacteria from the gut. So they can. The harmful bacteria that cause disease repeatedly get themselves doused with antibacterial drugs during the course of their long journeys through one person after another. The fact that they have survived these repeated drug attacks suggests they are resistant to them.

The normal intestinal bacteria give no cause to get themselves treated in this way, with the result that the normal intestinal bacteria are not encouraged to become resistant to antibacterial drugs. Normally, there are 50 billion bacteria in each pound of human feces. These myriads of minute chemical factories not only manufacture vitamins for us, but they also work very hard to produce chemicals that discourage the invasion of their territory by outsiders. They themselves manufacture antibiotics.

When antibacterial drugs are prescribed to eradicate diarrhea-causing bacteria from the intestines, the harmful bacteria often remain unharmed, and only the useful normal bacterial residents of our intestines get killed. The field is thus cleared for the invaders.

Often, the diarrhea is not cleared up until the course of the antibiotic is finished, or until the patient forgets to take his pills. If as occasionally happens, the invading bacteria are virulent and the beneficial residents are all exterminated, the patient is sped into his coffin almost as quickly as are his intestinal contents into a bedpan.

Sulphonamides, the earliest of the antibacterial drugs, were introduced into medicine during the late 1930s. Fifteen years later, practically all the diarrhea-causing bacteria had become resistant to sulphonamides. Nevertheless, the sulphonamides are still commonly prescribed as a treatment for diarrhea, and their manufacturers still advertise them in medical journals as useful for this purpose.

Aspirin

For feverish colds, doctors usually prescribe a simple analgesic. Two aspirins, a hot drink, and bed rest is perhaps the most frequently prescribed of all treatment regimes.

Aspirin makes one feel better and it reduces fever, but the true effect of aspirin on recovery has yet to be determined. Americans buy 6,500 tons of aspirin annually. Apart from causing gastric irritation and occasional bleeding, all this swallowed aspirin seems to cause remarkably few undesirable effects.

For young children, however, aspirin can be dangerous. In one three-year period, 79 youngsters were admitted to a Glasgow hospital with aspirin poisoning. Sixty-seven of these children had been accidentally poisoned; two died. The poisoning of the other 12 children was due to treatment overdoses; of these, six died. In the United States, aspirin accounts for 20 percent of all cases of poisoning in children under five years of age.

Phenacetin

Aspirin is a relatively safe drug; but phenacetin, a common

constituent of the more expensive proprietary brands of pain killers, is not so safe. In 1953, in a Swedish town in which a certain doctor had generally prescribed phenacetin, the death rate from kidney failure was more than three times that in a town of comparable size. Once the harmful effect of phenacetin upon kidneys was suspected, other cases of kidney damage due to this drug were soon reported.

A study of the pill-swallowing habits of 181 patients consecutively admitted to one mental hospital showed that 16 of them had each consumed during their lives more than two pounds of aspirin or phenacetin. These 16 patients were found to have a significantly higher incidence of dyspepsia, urinary symptoms, and kidney impairment.

Common pain-killers when taken regularly do not only kill pain. In Britain alone, about 75 deaths due to kidney failure are suspected of having been caused by the habitual use of phenacetin, according to a report made to the British Committee on the Safety of Drugs. These reported deaths most certainly are only the tip of the iceberg.

The Center for Drug Information of the U.S. Department of Health, Education, and Welfare has managed to pick up only a chip of this iceberg. A computer-assisted search of its records revealed only one death suspected from this cause. Since it is likely that several hundreds of such deaths occur in the United States each year, this particular government agency does not appear to be very astute at determining the lethal effects of many drugs that Americans use. Such effects are easily mistaken for natural diseases. It took more than 80 years of clinical use before the dangers of phenacetin were recognized. The use of this drug is now banned in some countries.

Treatment is nearly always assumed to be good until proved otherwise—and this takes some proving. Sir William Gull, the great 19th-century English physician who was disenchanted by the claims of success for the innumerable treatments for rheumatic fever, decided to expose human gullibility. So he published a paper extolling the virtues of mint as a cure for rheumatic fever. Other doctors, misunderstanding his purpose, prescribed a treatment of mint water, and for several years, mint water remained the fashionable cure for rheumatic fever. Many treatments continue to be popular simply because no one stops to question just how effective they really are.

Scientific Medicine

It would be grossly unjust to suggest that doctors and their treatments never do good. When doctors do use their expertise intelligently, they can be useful. The complex chemical structures and reactions that comprise a living organism are like those of a Rolls Royce engine. Even a Rolls can develop problems that require corrections by skilled mechanics.

Once doctors understand the machinery of the human body, they can become very adept, on occasion, at repairing its breakdowns. The body's need for minute spare parts—vitamins and the essential minerals—is now well understood. By assuring their adequate supply, doctors have been able to cure —and even better—to prevent a host of deficiency diseases.

Sometimes, doctors can replace defective or missing components of the body's machinery. The treatment of diabetes is an example of such a replacement. This disease develops when the pancreas stops producing insulin. Once this mechanism was understood, it became possible to replace the missing insulin by regular injections of this hormone. Health is then restored.

It is a simple matter to stop a Rolls Royce engine from working; a wrench thrown into the works will do it at once. The same is true of a living organism. Doctors now have all sorts of spanners that they can throw into the works of a living creature. Some of these monkey wrenches are particularly useful since they are relatively harmless to us, but quite destructive to the organism that has invaded a human body. Penicillin is usually quite harmless to humans, but that drug destroys certain bacteria by blocking the building up of chemicals in their cell walls. Chloroquin kills the malarial parasite, but not us.

It is substances such as these that have done so much to change the face of modern treatment. Nevertheless, these drugs do not work by magic, but by interfering with the vital chemical processes of life. Used unwisely, they are as likely to harm us as they are to harm our microscopic enemies.

While scientific advances have rendered some treatments more useful, these new treatments have also led us into trouble. Early treatments were exalted even when most of them did not work. With the discovery of the wonder drugs such as penicil-

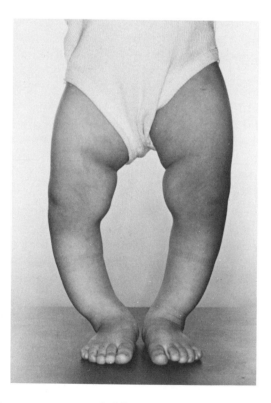

Not so long ago, many children had bandy legs because of rickets, and grew up to be deformed adults. Today, thanks to improved nutrition and maternity care, this disease is very rare.

lin, treatment has become a cult; we have become votaries of the colored pill. Unfortunately for the practice of good medicine, we are worshiping the wrong god. Treatment is not what keeps such large numbers of us alive and well; it is good preventive medicine and improved hygiene that does so.

Unostentatious departments of public health are what make the Western countries healthful places to live in. Compared to most other governmental agencies, these departments spend comparatively small sums of public money. Yet these health agencies work wonders for us. By insuring that sewage is kept out of the water supply, these bureaus have abolished typhoid and cholera. By establishing vaccination against small-pox, whooping cough, diphtheria, tuberculosis, and poliomyelitis, these agencies have all but eliminated these serious diseases.

Rickets was once a common cause of bow-leggedness and dwarfing. Scantly more than half a century ago, 80 percent of the school children in the working-class East End of London had rickets. In Philadelphia, a century ago, 25 percent of all children under the age of five were ricketic. Today, maternity and child welfare clinics help maintain the health of pregnant mothers and infants, and rickets is seldom seen.

When health cranks allow it, public health departments add fluoride to the water supply in areas where its natural concentration is low. This element helps our children's teeth to resist decay. Government enforcement of pure food and drug laws means the food we buy is healthful. Enforcement of industrial safety laws limits the exposure of workers to harmful substances. For example, silica no longer kills miners by the thousands, nor does mercury make hatters mad.

In addition to the public health departments' effective work in the prevention of disease, the real reasons why most of us remain alive and kicking are the more equal distribution of wealth, which has reduced killing poverty; and the improvements in contraceptive techniques, which have reduced the number of unwanted children with their above-average mortality rates.

Treatment of established disease is a most inefficient way of insuring survival in good health. In terms of lives saved, *preventive medicine has been much more successful.* Could prevention be rendered still more effective?

Certainly, pollution remains a major source of ill health. But apart from a much needed heavy attack on our chimneys, our car exhaust systems, and on our industrial effluent, there is little more that our public health departments can do to increase the level of our good health.

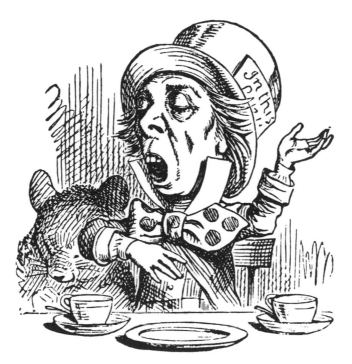

The Mad Hatter from Alice's Adventures in Wonderland *is, sadly, based in fact. Nineteenth-century hatters were often driven mad and made to tremble by the mercury which they used to make hats pliable. In the United States, this disease was known as the "Danbury Shakes," after the Connecticut hat-making city.*

SOURCES

Adams, B. G., Horder, E. J., Horder, J. P., et al: "Patients Receiving Barbiturates in an Urban General Practice." *Journal of the College of General Practitioners,* 12 24 (1966).

Anderson, G. W., and Rondean, J. C.: "Absence of Tonsils as a Factor in the Development of Bulbar Poliomyelitis." *Journal of the American Medical Association,* 155 1123 (1954).

Armitage, S. G.: "The Effects of Barbiturates on the Behaviour of Rat Offspring." *Journal of Comparative Physiology and Psychology,* 45 146 (1952).

Bakwin, Harry: "Pseudodoxia Pediatrica." *New England Journal of Medicine,* 232 691 (1945).

Bellville, R. E., and Frazer, H. F.: "Tolerance to Some Effects of Barbiturates." *Journal of Pharmacology and Experimental Therapeutics,* 120 469 (1957).

British Medical Association and Pharmaceutical Society of Great Britain: *The British National Formulary.* London: BMA, 1963.

British Medical Journal: "Tonsils and Adenoids." 2 698 (1963).

————: "Further Doubts about Oral Contraceptives." 1 252 (1970).

Brokbank, William: *Ancient Therapeutic Arts.* London: Heinemann, 1954.

Brunton, Sir Thomas Lauder: *Lectures on the Action of Medicines.* London: Macmillan, 1897.

Cochrane, A. L.: *Effectiveness and Efficiency.* London: Nuffield Provincial Hospitals Trust, 1972.

Comfort, Alex: *The Anxiety Makers.* London: Thomas Nelson, 1967.

Community Health Center Project: The Community Health Center in Canada (The Hastings Report). Canada 1972.

Craig, J. O., Ferguson, I. C., and Syme, J.: "Infants, Toddlers and Aspirin." *British Medical Journal,* 1 757 (1966).

Dunlop, Sir Derek: "Drugs: Their Uses and Abuses." *Veterinary Record,* 85 424 (1969).

Fanconi, Von G., and Botsztejn, A.: "Die Feersche Krankheit (Akrodynie) und Quecksilbermedikation." *Helvetica Paediatrica Acta,* 3 264 (1948).

Ferguson, Margaret: "A Study of the Social and Economic Factors in the Causation of Rickets." (National Health Insurance Joint Committee. Medical Research Council.) London: Her Majesty's Stationery Office, 1918.

Fry, John: "Are All T's and A's Really Necessary?" *British Medical Journal,* 1 124 (1957).

Gaddum, J. H.: *Pharmacology.* London: Oxford University Press. 1959.

Garrison, F. M.: *An Introduction to the History of Medicine.* Philadelphia and London: W. B. Saunders Co., 1929.

Graves, R. J.: *Clinical Lectures on the Practice of Medicine.* London: New Sydenham Society, 1884.

Hale-White, Sir William: *Great Doctors of the 19th Century.* London: Edward Arnold & Co., 1935.

Holt, L. E., McIntosh, R., and Barnett, H. L.: *Pediatrics.* New York: Appleton-Century-Crofts, Inc., 1962.

Hurwitz, Natalie: "Intensive Hospital Monitoring of Adverse Reactions to Drugs." *British Medical Journal,* 1 53 (1969).

Jessner, Lucie, Blom, Gaston E., and Waldfogel, Samuel: "Emotional Implications of Tonsillectomy and Adenoidectomy in Children." In *The Psychoanalytic Study of the Child.* Vol. 7. New York: International Universities Press, 1952.

Laurence, D. R.: *Clinical Pharmacology.* London: J. & A. Churchill, 1966.

Lave, L. B., and Seskin, E. P.: "Air Pollution and Human Health." *Science,* **169** 723 (1970).

Levy, David: "Psychic Trauma of Operations in Children." *American Journal of Diseases of Children,* **69** 7 (1945).

Luce, G. G., and Segal, J.: *Sleep.* London: Heinemann, 1967.

Ministry of Health: "Deaths from Tonsillectomy." In *Report on Hospital In-Patient Inquiry for the Year 1961.* London: Her Majesty's Stationery Office, 1962.

Murray, R. M., Timbury, G. C., and Linton, A. L.: "Analgesic

Abuse in Psychiatric Patients." *Lancet,* **1** 1303 (1970).

Oswald, I., and Priest, R. G.: "Five Weeks to Escape the Sleeping Pill Habit." *British Medical Journal,* **2** 1093 (1965).

Pearson, Gerald H. J.: "Effects of Operative Procedures on the Emotional Life of the Child." *American Journal of Diseases of Children,* **62** 716 (1941).

Rovinsky, Joseph J.: "Preliminary Experience with a Permissive Abortion Statute." *Obstetrics and Gynecology,* **38** (3) 333 (1971).

Schimmel, E. M.: "The Hazards of Hospitalization." *Annals of Internal Medicine,* **60** 100 (1964).

Seidl, L. G., Thornton, G. F., Smith, J. W., et al: "Studies on the Epidemiology of Adverse Drug Reactions: (3) Reactions in Patients on a General Medical Service." *Johns Hopkins Hospital Bulletin,* **119** 299 (1966).

Skinner, H. A.: *The Origin of Medical Terms.* Baltimore: Williams and Wilkins Co., 1961.

U. S. Bureau of Census: *Statistical Abstract of the U.S.A.* Washington, D.C., Government Printing Office, 1971.

U. S. Department of Health, Education, and Welfare: "Tabulations of 1969 Reports." *Bulletin of the Poison Control Center, National Clearing House,* Sept.–Oct. 1970.

Vianna, Nicholas J., Greenwald, Peter, and Davies, J. N. P.: "Tonsillectomy and Hodgkin's Disease: The Lymph Barrier." *Lancet,* **1** 431 (1971).

Warkany, J., and Hubbard, D. M.: "Mercury in the Urine of Children with Acrodynia." *Lancet,* **1** 829 (1948).

Weick, M. T.: "A History of Rickets in the United States." *American Journal of Clinical Nutrition,* **20** 1234 (1967).

Werboff, J., and Kesner, R.: "Learning Deficit of Rat Offspring After Administrations of Tranquilizing Drugs to the Mothers." *Nature,* **197** 106 (1964).

Wolman, I. J.: "Tonsillectomy and Adenoidectomy: An Analysis of a Nationwide Inquiry into Prevailing Medical Practices." *Quarterly Review of Pediatrics,* **II** 109 (1956).

Patient, Heal Thyself

Government laws are concerned with public health. But how can our individual good health be further improved? The answer is simple, though perhaps discomforting. We ourselves are best suited to accomplish improvement.

If the overweight ate less, the drinkers drank less, the smokers stopped smoking, and everyone took a little more exercise, we would as a group gain many more years of healthful life. We would, by virtue of such a program, eradicate more disease than we can possibly do by supplying the best and the most expensive of modern treatments for the cure of disease. Even if we abolished doctors and their treatments, the general life expectancy would still increase, and of course treatment itself bumps off quite a lot of us each year.

I believe that doctors, by being so good-naturedly optimistic about how they can help everybody, do the community a disservice. People are lulled into believing that health can be left to the physicians.

The 10 leading causes of death in the so-called advanced countries are today: heart disease; cancer; stroke; physical accidents; flu, pneumonia and bronchitis; diabetes; birth injuries; cirrhosis of the liver; congenital malformations; and suicide. Cigarettes, alcohol, physical inactivity, and overeating are major contributors to the incidence of several of these killers.

Cigarettes

Smoking increases our chances of dying from three major causes of death: chronic bronchitis, coronary thrombosis, and cancer. People who smoke 25 cigarettes or more a day are 30 times more likely to die of lung cancer and six times more likely to die of chronic bronchitis than are non-smokers. Men between the ages of 45 and 54 who smoke more than 10 cigarettes a day are three times more likely to die of coronary heart disease than are non-smokers. The more cigarettes a person smokes, the more often is he sick. Those who smoke 40 cigarettes a day are, on average, absent nearly twice as much from work as are their non-smoking associates.

Smoking has increased greatly over the past 50 years, and so have the diseases that it causes. In England, in 1900, there were 273 registered deaths from lung cancer; now there are over 30,000 each year. Today, cancer of the lung accounts for over a third of all deaths from cancer. Moreover, the incidence of some other cancers besides those of the lung is also increased by smoking.

Cigarettes are probably responsible for the fact that the life expectancy of middle-aged Englishmen is no better today than it was 50 years ago. It is not for nothing that cigarettes are called coffin nails. Three-quarters of the men and half the women of Britain now smoke. Some 44 million Americans buy their own personal pollution kits of tobacco.

Alcohol

No one knows how much illness and how many deaths are attributable to alcohol. The heavy drinker averages four times as much absence from work as does the non-alcoholic. Alcoholism certainly kills. Due to malnutrition, cirrhosis of the liver, pneumonia, and suicide, an alcoholic's life expectancy is 10 to 12 years shorter than that of the non-alcoholic.

About 350,000 people in Britain, or 1 percent of the population, are alcoholics. One fourth of these people show mental and physical deterioration. As a group, Americans drink the British under the table. At least 4 percent of adult Americans are alcoholic, and some 300 million dollars are spent every year on advertising campaigns which encourage them to be so. Although dedicated communists once regarded alcoholism as a disease of capitalism, Russia's figures for alcoholism match those of the United States.

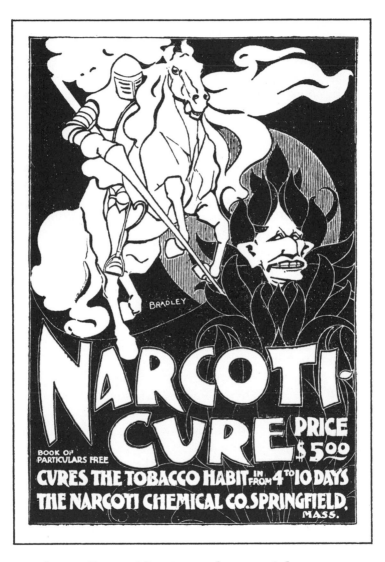

Slaying Demon Nicotine at the turn of the century.

Alcohol causes accidents. Numerous studies in North America prove that in more than half the deaths caused by traffic accidents, alcohol is the true malefactor. Nearly three-quarters of a million people have been killed on the American roads in the last quarter century.

In England, in 1967, when the breathalyzer frightened the inebriated off the roads, there was a reduction of one in seven road deaths compared to the previous year; 1,152 fewer people died. In the United States, the Chicago courts made a highly publicized threat to award a seven-day jail sentence to everyone convicted of drunk driving during the Christmas and New Year holiday period of 1971. It resulted in over a thousand less traffic accidents and 64 percent fewer road deaths than during the same time period of the previous year.

Drunken drivers are not the only offenders. A survey made of 64 injured pedestrians taken to a Manchester, England, hospital between midnight and six in the morning showed that they all were intoxicated.

Inactivity and Overeating

Too much food and too little exercise also takes years off our lives. Obesity is associated with an increased incidence of several serious diseases—heart disease, diabetes, bronchitis, high blood pressure.

Life insurance companies, by recording the height, weight, and build of their many millions of clients and then watching to see how long they take to die, are able to determine those weights which, for individuals of varying heights and builds, are associated with the greatest longevity. These weights they call desirable. Figures published by the Metropolitan Life Insurance Company show that American men who are 10 percent or more above their desirable weight have an excess mortality of nearly one-half. Women are biologically tougher than men; they carry their weight better. But even for women, each surplus pound is a small stepping stone to the grave.

Nearly 50 percent of American men and almost 40 percent

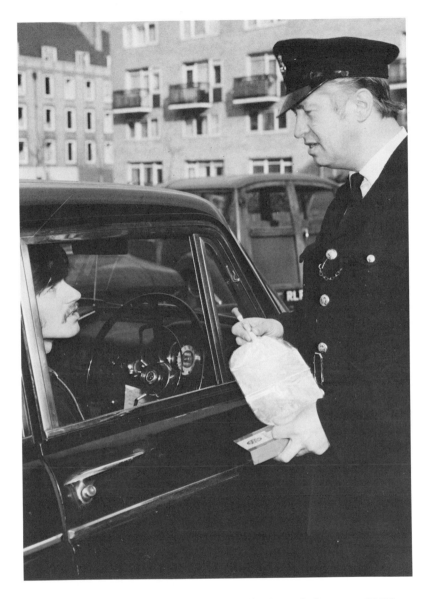

*In England, the introduction of the breathalyzer in 1967
frightened the inebriated off the roads. In that year, road
deaths fell by 14 percent.*

of American women between the ages of 30 and 39 are more than 10 percent overweight.

Doctors Defeated

Medicine has little help to offer for self-induced conditions of ill health. Chronic bronchitis follows an inexorable course of breathless discomfort. Despite the most modern and most expensive means of medical intervention, people with coronary thrombosis continue to die. In fact, it has been suggested that intensive care units, with all their electronic equipment, are actually frightening patients to death; a man with a coronary may have a better chance to survive if he stays in the quiet and comfort of his own home.

Surgery is the only treatment that offers any chance of long-time survival for people with lung cancer, but only about one-fifth of all cases are suitable for operation. Of those who undergo surgery for cancer of the lung, two-thirds will die within three years.

Psychiatrists are also singularly unsuccessful at stopping people from drinking. The World Health Organization expert committee on mental health defines the criterion for cure of an alcoholic as two years of total abstinence. Only 18 percent of 50 alcoholics treated at the Mecca of English psychiatry, the Maudsley Hospital, met this criterion.

A very small number of specialized hospitals on both sides of the Atlantic carefully select those alcoholics who are most likely to benefit by three to four months of intensive treatment in hospital. These hospitals have cure rates of about one third. The spontaneous cure rate for alcoholics who stop drinking by themselves is about 10 percent. For the average alcoholic in the average hospital, it is doubtful if the cure rate is any better than that of spontaneous cure. Since many doctors themselves believe that problems can be cured by chemicals, it may be that doctors are not good for boozers. So far doctors have had more success at causing addiction than at curing it.

Doctors have never had much success with the obese.

Eating less requires resolution; treatments are much more popular. Today, amphetamines and other addictive stimulants are in vogue. But these diet pills are not very effective at making people thin. John Yudkin, professor of dietetics at London Uni-

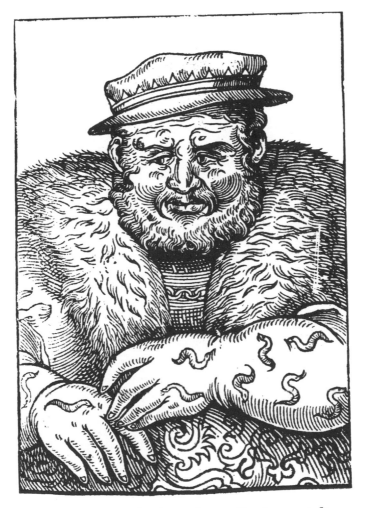

Leeches were once the doctor's standby for most diseases. They were an obvious treatment for the overweight. As the leeches grew fatter, the patient grew thinner.

versity, treated one group of obese patients with pills and another group without pills. Those treated without the reducing pills lost more weight. They were not waiting for the pills to work.

Medical Researches

Three types of research are popular in medical science: drug firms search for drugs; clinicians search for new treatments; and pure scientists search for new basic knowledge.

Drug companies are not charitable institutions; they are not supposed to be. They are sometimes responsible for some excellent research work, and they help finance medical conferences and periodicals. But drug companies do not exist solely for the good of our health. Like breweries and tobacco

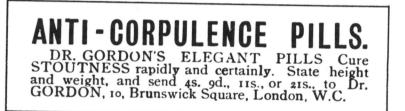

ANTI-CORPULENCE PILLS.
DR. GORDON'S ELEGANT PILLS Cure STOUTNESS rapidly and certainly. State height and weight, and send 4s. 9d., 11s., or 21s., to Dr. GORDON, 10, Brunswick Square, London, W.C.

Fat people prefer pills to exercise, for pills can be eaten. Dr. Grey offered electric pills, Dr. Gordon offered "elegant" ones. Today, doctors recommend amphetamines and other addictive stimulants.

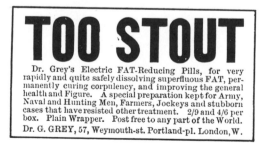

TOO STOUT
Dr. Grey's Electric FAT-Reducing Pills, for very rapidly and quite safely dissolving superfluous FAT, permanently curing corpulency, and improving the general health and Figure. A special preparation kept for Army, Naval and Hunting Men, Farmers, Jockeys and stubborn cases that have resisted other treatment. 2/9 and 4/6 per box. Plain Wrapper. Post free to any part of the World.
Dr. G. GREY, 57, Weymouth-st. Portland-pl. London, W.

companies, they are commercial enterprises devoted to making a profit. Our colds, our aches, our pains, our mental discomforts, and our insomnia are their gold mines.

Drug companies, breweries, and tobacco companies all exploit our predilection for addictive chemicals. The most profitable drugs are generally those which are gently addictive. Such drugs are, after all, assured of a regular and enthusiastic clientele. Drug companies would like everyone to believe that their products work only wonders; but in some countries, they are now obliged by law to confess in their literature the recognized dangers of their products.

Clinicians are interested in what they can do, not in what they cannot do. No doctor wins himself a reputation if he cannot cure diseases. Doctors offer treatments—that is their stock in trade. The disadvantages of their treatments are somehow overlooked.

A team studying the incidence of adverse drug reaction at Johns Hopkins Hospital reported that their survey of a group of 150 patients turned up four times as many adverse drug reactions as were reported during the same period by all the rest of the doctors associated with the 1,100-bed hospital.

If doctors and the press reported the adverse effects of other drugs with even a quarter of the enthusiasm with which they report the side effects of "the Pill"—of which they often disapprove—a great many people would become anxious about the effects of the medicines we so enthusiastically swallow. There would be a nasty recession in the pharmaceutical industry.

In England, doctors are requested to report adverse drug reactions to the Committee on the Safety of Drugs, but they are not very conscientious about doing so. It is not comfortable for a doctor to admit that his prescribed medication turned little Johnnie blue; it is easier to regard blueness as an unusual manifestation of Johnnie's disease.

Doctors in the United States and Canada have a similar system of reporting. The doctor in charge of the Canadian program thinks his service would be doing well if one-half of

1 percent of all suspected adverse drug reactions were actually reported. Precisely because the adverse effects of drugs usually go unreported, it is difficult to know exactly how dangerous many drugs are.

Pure theoretical scientists search for new basic knowledge of the science of man; few are interested in treatment or in its effects. The disadvantages of our drugs are thus quietly forgotten.

Patients are even more predisposed than doctors to unquestioningly accept the usefulness of treatments. Several studies have shown that about 30 percent of patients with physical illnesses and 40 percent of patients with psychiatric illnesses say they feel better on being given completely inert substances or placebos. Such gullibility makes the introduction of any new treatment easy, for roughly a third of all recipients will claim that the treatment works even though it is only colored water.

Charlatans often achieve remarkable therapeutic successes by their ability to convince patients of the certainty of recovery. Though such cures have their uses, they are perhaps gained at the expense of increasing the patient's dependency upon his doctor, and diminishing his own stature as a person.

Science Makes Things Happen

Even when powerful modern drugs are used sensibly, such drugs can yield unanticipated results. The treatment of diabetes can serve as an example. Insulin lowers the blood sugar of a diabetic and returns him to health; but insulin has the big disadvantage that it must be given by injection. Scientists then discovered that the sulfonylureas, which can be taken by mouth, will also lower the diabetic's blood sugar. These new drugs have now been in use for some 15 years.

Tolbutamide, a proprietary preparation of one of the sulfonylureas, is most commonly used. A follow-up study published in 1970 shows not only that the combination of diet and Tolbutamide is no more effective than diet alone, but that

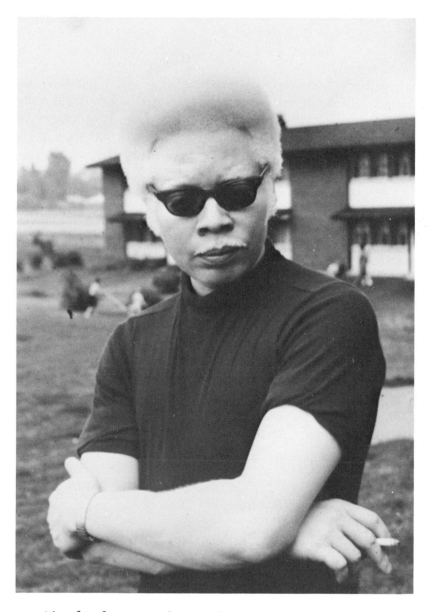

After his doctor put him on the sedative Doriden, this once jet-black Negro turned white and his hair turned blond. This is but one of a myriad of treatment surprises.

after eight years of trial, the death rate from cardiovascular disease in those diabetics who received Tolbutamide was two and one half times higher than among those who had received only a placebo.

Nobody had suspected that Tolbutamide might have an adverse effect on the heart. About 800,000 Americans take Tolbutamide every day. In 1969, sales of the drug totaled 50 million dollars. Yet one study claims that 8,000 Americans have died prematurely each year because of the use of Tolbutamide.

Powerful and biologically active drugs certainly have their uses. Even a drug with a 50 percent mortality record would still be useful if it cured a disease that was 100 percent fatal. It would be useful as long as doctors did not prescribe such a drug to people who did not have a fatal disease in the first place.

We will, no doubt, continue to clamor for medicines, and the pharmaceutical industry will continue to produce a lot of new ones, and doctors will continue enthusiastically to prescribe them. It is only when the birth of little monsters follows the use of a new brand of sleeping tablet, or a new pill turns black men white, or a rash of unexpected deaths occurs among enthusiastic users of pain killers, that the untoward effects of many drugs are forced upon our notice.

The continuing development of new drugs by the pharmaceutical industry will do more good than harm, only if the medical profession organizes research to discover exactly what these drugs are doing to their patients; and having found this out, if they then prescribe these drugs sensibly. At present, the medical profession too often relies on the claims made by the drug companies. The medical profession seldom organizes such research, and seldom does it use new drugs prudently.

SOURCES

American Diabetic Association: "The University Group Diabetes Program." *Diabetes,* **19** Supplement 2 (1970).

Beecher, H. K.: "The Powerful Placebo." *Journal of the American Medical Association,* **154** 1602 (1955).

Borrie, J.: *Lung Cancer: Surgery and Survival.* New York: Appleton-Century-Crofts, Inc., 1965.

Campbell, E. O'F.: "Alcohol Involvement in Fatal Motor Vehicle Accidents." *Modern Medicine of Canada,* **24** (4) 35 (1969); *Modern Medicine of Canada,* **26** (7) 7 (1971).

Cassie, A. B., and Allan, W. R.: "Alcohol and Road Traffic Accidents." *British Medical Journal,* **2** 1668 (1961).

Commission of Inquiry into the Non-Medical Use of Drugs: *Treatment.* Information Canada, Ottawa: 1972.

Craddock, Denis: *Obesity and Its Management.* Edinburgh: E. & S. Livingston, 1969.

Davies, D. L., Shepherd, M., and Myers, E.: "Two Years Prognosis of Fifty Alcoholics After Treatment in Hospital." *Quarterly Journal of Studies on Alcoholism,* **17** 485 (1956).

Doll, R., and Hill, Sir A. B.: "Mortality in Relation to Smoking, Ten Years Observation of British Doctors." *British Medical Journal,* **1** 1460 (1964).

Franks, Cyril M.: "Alcoholism." In *Symptoms of Psychopathology.* Ed. Charles G. Costello. New York: John Wiley & Sons, Inc., 1970.

Gardham, A. J., and Davies, D. R.: *The Operations of Surgery.* London: J. & A. Churchill, 1969.

Glatt, M. M.: "An Alcoholic Unit in a Mental Hospital." *Lancet,* **2** 397 (1959).

Hammond, E. C.: "Smoking in Relation to the Death Rates of One Million Men and Women. Epidemiological Approaches to the Study of Cancer and Other Diseases." (U. S. Public Health Services, National Cancer Institute Monograph 19) Bethesda, Md.: 1966.

Hill, M. J., and Blane, H. T.: "Evaluation of Psychotherapy with

Alcoholics: A Critical Review." *Quarterly Journal of Studies on Alcoholism,* **28** 76 (1967).

Irons, Evelyn: "The White Negroes." *The Sunday Times Magazine* (London), Jan. 17, 1971.

Kessel, N., and Grossman, G.: "Suicide in Alcoholics." *British Medical Journal,* **2** 1671 (1961).

―――― and Walton, Henry: *Alcoholism.* London: Penguin Books, 1969.

Laurence, D. R.: *Clinical Pharmacology.* London: J. & A. Churchill, 1966.

McCarthy, Raymond G.: "Alcoholism Rates." In *Alcohol Education for Classroom and Community.* Ed. Raymond G. McCarthy. New York: McGraw Hill, 1964.

M.D. of Canada: "The Egregious Quacks." **13** (3) 75 (1972).

Metropolitan Life Insurance Co.: "Mortality from Accidents by Age and Sex." *Statistical Bulletin,* **52** 6 (1971).

―――― : "Overweight. Its Prevention and Significance." *Statistical Bulletin,* 1960.

Pincherle, G., and Wright, H. B.: "Screening in the Early Diagnosis and Prevention of Cardiovascular Disease." *Journal of the College of General Practitioners,* **13** 280 (1967).

Registrar General: *Statistical Review of England and Wales for the Year 1967.* London: Her Majesty's Stationery Office, 1968.

Royal College of Physicians: *Smoking and Health: Summary and Report on Smoking in Relation to Cause of Cancer of the Lung and Other Diseases.* Toronto: McClelland and Stewart, Ltd., 1962.

Seidl, L. G., Thornton, G. F., and Cluff, L. E.: "Epidemiological Study of Adverse Drug Reactions." *American Journal of Public Health,* **55** 1170 (1965).

Smith, David J.: "Absenteeism and 'Presenteeism' in Industry." *Archives of Environmental Health,* **21** 670 (1970).

Thompson, Vernon C.: *Clinical Surgery.* Ed. Charles Rob and Rodney Smith. London: Butterworth, 1965.

Toronto Daily Star: "U. S. Probing Anti-Diabetic Pill, Feared Cause of Early Deaths." May 22, 1970.

Trice, H. M., and Belasco, J. A.: "Patterns of Absenteeism Among Problem Drinkers." *Management Review,* **56** 55 (1967).

U. S. Bureau of Census: *Statistical Abstract of the U.S.A.* Washington, D. C.: Government Printing Office, 1971.

World Health Organization, Expert Committee on Mental Health: *Report on the First Session of the Alcoholism Subcommittee* (Technical Report No. 42) WHO, 2 (1951).

Yudkin, J. I.: "The Treatment of Obesity." *Medical Press,* **246** (3) 64 (1961).

Doctors for the Mind

Hence, loathed Melancholy
Of Cerberus, and blackest Midnight born,
In Stygian cave forlorn,
'Mongst horrid shapes, and shrieks and sights unholy.

JOHN MILTON

Separate studies made of the incidence of mental disorder in the skyscraper jungle of midtown Manhattan and of the incidence of mental disorder in a quiet rural seaside county in Nova Scotia reached the same conclusions. One-fifth of each of the two populations had mental symptoms severe enough to cause significant impairment of functioning. A further three-fifths had some symptoms of emotional impairment. Only one-fifth of each population were found to be psychiatrically quite well.

In another study, it was found that between one-tenth and one-fifth of the patient population of 46 doctors in general practice in Greater London were mentally disturbed.

Mental illness is diagnosed either when the patient complains of uncomfortable mental symptoms or when his behavior is considered by others to be abnormal or unacceptable. Psychiatry is the branch of medicine that is concerned with mental illness; and psychiatry is undoubtedly the fastest growing branch in medicine.

Mind and Matter

The brain is the organ of the mind. Its chemical and electrical activity is associated with consciousness. Although the functioning of the brain must be incredibly complicated, its basic design is quite simple.

Information in the form of nerve impulses is continuously fed to the brain from the sense receptors. It is estimated that about a million information impulses reach the brain at any one time. And the brain processes this information.

Nerve impulses are then sent from the brain to the muscles of the body. These muscles react. Out of this simple mechanism are elaborated all the complexities of speech and behavior.

A child withdraws his hand from a hot coal. This is an inborn pattern of behavior. But he learns that glowing coals hurt: he no longer wants to play with them. Similarly, a child learns ways of responding to people, to situations, and to those internal events which, like fear and excitement, happen within himself. It is the sum of all these responses that will determine his behavior.

The ways in which an individual has habitually learned to respond to things, to people, to situations, and to his biological urges have made him the sort of person he is. We learn to respond to new situations with interest or with anxiety. We learn to respond to other people with warmth or with suspicion. We learn ways of responding to our own anxiety. Some of us learn to tolerate large amounts of anxiety; others, when faced with even some small worries, just go to pieces.

What then is mental illness? If one experiences uncomfortable mental symptoms, or if one's behavior becomes disturbed to the extent that others say he is mentally ill, then there can be only two possible explanations.

The first is that the disturbed individual has not learned to respond to people, and to situations, and to his own feelings in ways that others regard as satisfactory. He has not learned to cope with life. He has not learned useful "life lessons."

The second explanation is that his brain is not working properly. The machinery with which he receives, stores, and processes information is malfunctioning. He can no longer respond in appropriate ways. Of course, it is possible, and it frequently happens, that his behavior is disturbed for both of the foregoing reasons.

Life Lessons

Why do people fail to learn their life lessons? Probably for much the same reasons a child fails to learn his school lessons: either he is a dull child, or he is not interested in learning them, or his teacher is a failure.

The bright learn life lessons more easily than the stupid. A group of school children with IQ's of 140 or above suffered less mental illness as adults than the average. The old Victorian idea of "early to ripen, early to rot"—that the bright child is the most susceptible to mental derangement—has not withstood sociological investigation. Conversely, the incidence of so-called mental illness is highest in the lowest economic class; and, in general, members of this class have an IQ lower than the average.

Some people do not learn life lessons because they are not interested in doing so. A man, for instance, who prefers his mother to his wife is unlikely to learn to be an adequate husband. For others, learning is made difficult because they are inadequately taught. It is difficult to learn to be a caring human being from parents who are uncaring, or to learn honesty in a household of crooks.

A schoolboy who through indifference, incompetence, or poor teaching fails to make college is not usually regarded as mentally ill. A man who fails to learn his life lessons often is. But is this extension of the meaning of illness useful? Is it useful, for instance, to regard as sick the addict who uses drugs because he has not learned to face the anxiety of coping with life?

More and more, society and psychiatry are coming to regard addiction as a mental illness. This attitude turns a man who has a lot of learning to do into a patient, who can then sit back and wait for his doctor to get him better. He stays sick, and his doctor stays useless.

Behavior may be disturbed because the brain is not functioning properly. A return to normal behavior will be achieved only if and when the defect is corrected.

Brain Diseases

In 1913, Hideyo Noguchi demonstrated the presence of the spirochete of syphilis in the brains of patients dying from general paralysis of the insane. Only 50 years ago, it was estimated that one in six Americans who became mentally ill had brain syphilis. In fact, among men of high school or college education, brain syphilis caused more "mental illness" than all other causes combined.

Although the progress of brain syphilis can now be halted by treatment, the damaged brain can never be restored to normal, and the patient remains insane. But once the cause of the disease was understood, it became possible—by screening all hospital patients for syphilis, tracing all contacts, and treating all cases early, and through such measures as premarital medical requirements—to make brain syphilis a very rare disease. This splendid result must be regarded as one of the few shining examples of good "psychiatry"—although, in reality, psychiatrists had very little to do with it.

The brain, like other organs of the body, is subject to a great number of disease processes. Injury, hardening of its arteries, chemicals, drugs, and viruses can all interfere with normal brain functioning. When the brain is diseased, behavior and the "mind" usually become disturbed.

The human mind is infinitely variable; but the kinds of alteration in its functioning caused by brain disease are limited: alteration of consciousness, changes of mood, loss of drive, alteration of perception, interruption of normal processes of thought and expression, disturbances of memory,

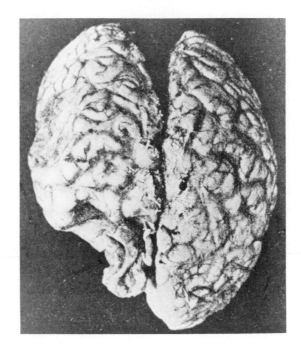

Once the spirochaete of syphilis has nibbled at a man's brain, his behavior becomes disturbed. This photograph illustrates a brain destroyed by syphilis.

and the appearance of firmly held false beliefs.

Illnesses in which a disease of the brain interferes with normal mental functioning are classed as mental illnesses. This is a misnomer. The patient has mental symptoms but not mental illness; the brain is sick, not the mind. One does not expect psychotherapy to put color into the cheeks of a girl with an iron deficiency anemia, nor should one expect psychotherapy to cure a depressed and deluded woman who has a deficiency of thyroid hormone. Only thyroid tablets will do so.

Disturbed behavior is like a wrong answer from a computer. The computer has either been inadequately programmed, or it has internal misconnections that prevent it from working properly. A computer is attended by two kinds of experts: a programmer who feeds appropriate information into it; and an electronic engineer who takes care of its machinery. For the mentally disturbed human, the two jobs are performed by one man, the psychiatrist. And the psychiatrist often ends up doing both jobs rather badly.

Before a useful treatment can be found for a disease, it is nearly always necessary to know the cause of the disease. Only on the luckiest of occasions have useful treatments been discovered by chance. The brain is by far the most complicated organ of the body; its study is made difficult because it is enclosed in a bony box. We still know very little about how the brain works, and how it can go wrong.

Seldom are psychiatrists good physicians. Only a minority of psychiatrists are interested in searching for possible causes of brain disease. For the most part, psychiatrists busy themselves either with symptomatic cures, or with helping their patients to understand why they behave as they do. As many of these symptomatic cures are of doubtful efficacy, and since nobody knows what really determines how we feel and how we behave, psychiatrists have not had very much success. "Fools," as the proverb says, "rush in where angels fear to tread." Psychiatrists, by and large, are not exactly hesitant.

Psychiatric Comfort

Hippocrates gave to medicine the motto "To cure sometimes; to relieve often; and to comfort always." In Greece, in the 5th century B.C., when disease meant a half-severed arm from a lance blow, or a festering tumor the size of an orange on the end of one's nose, such advice on professional conduct was obviously right and proper. But in the comfortable 20th century, when disease may mean a hangover or a family quarrel, such solicitude may no longer be useful.

To supply a healthy but disgruntled young wife with a bottle of pills may be a comfort to her; but that bottle probably does not help her family quarrels. There is nothing wrong with her brain. The pills, whatever they are, cannot be expected to improve its functioning; they can only interfere with its normality. This interference may help her to forget her problems and make her feel better; but the pills are not likely to make her behave any better. Indeed, because after she takes the drugs her brain will not work so well, more likely she will not cope so well.

Psychiatrists are hampered by a difficult problem. Much of the time, they cannot decide if disturbed behavior is due to a disorder of the brain or to faulty learning; this means that they do not really know how to set such behavior right.

Schizophrenia

Schizophrenia causes the most uncertainty. It is a common and serious disease the cause of which is not known, though some psychiatrists believe that mothers who make irrational and conflicting demands on their children, induce in their children this disease. For a child subject to conflicting demands, whose mother expects him to be independent and yet always do what he is told to do, insanity becomes a sane solution.

Other psychiatrists dismiss the "schizophrenogenic Mom" and believe the disease to be caused by a chemical, which when extracted from the schizophrenic's urine and stained, makes a pink spot on blotting paper. Other psychiatrists deem the pink spot to be just another red herring.

In fact, schizophrenia probably is not one disease but a hodgepodge of disorders all showing a similar configuration of mental symptoms. The majority of early cases recover spontaneously, though sometimes a person's personality is left impaired. Some people have repeated attacks; in others, the disease has an insidious onset and chronic course.

In any disease which always proves to be fatal, it is obvious whether a treatment is useful or not. If patients continue to die after its use, the conclusion is clear.

Where partial or complete recovery occurs spontaneously,

the usefulness of a treatment is much more difficult to assess. Sir William Gull used to annoy his colleagues by saying, "Medicines do most good when there is a tendency to recover without them." When recovery follows treatment, doctors, not unnaturally, like to take the credit.

There are two certainties in medicine: (1) The less effective the treatment for a disease, the greater will be the number of their variety; (2) irrational treatments usually do more harm than good. The treatment of schizophrenia is no exception. There are many treatments for it. Probably most of them are harmful.

Insulin Coma

Insulin coma treatment for schizophrenia was introduced into psychiatry in Berlin in 1932, and rapidly gained a reputation as *the* effective treatment. Expensive insulin units were established in all mental hospitals. Comas were induced in the schizophrenic patient every day, with the average course of treatment lasting six to eight weeks. Many patients were given several such courses.

In 1953, after practically every schizophrenic in Europe and many in North America had been subjected to insulin coma, Dr. H. Bourne published in the *Lancet* an article entitled "The Insulin Myth." Analyzing the studies that had been made of the results of this treatment, he pointed out their common fallacies, and he showed that insulin was not a useful treatment for schizophrenia.

The reception of his article was mixed. One friendly *Lancet* correspondent wrote:

> *Doctor Bourne has done well in destroying the myth of the cure of schizophrenia by insulin. Having treated schizophrenia for years by various methods, I have now no doubt that those who recovered after being treated by insulin recovered in spite of treatment, and not because of it; and I am relieved that*

I no longer submit my patients to a treatment so unpleasant, dangerous, and useless.

Four years later, Dr. B. Ackner and his colleagues published the results of a properly controlled study of insulin treatment. Half of a group of patients were treated by insulin coma, and the other half by barbiturate anesthesia. The same number of patients recovered in the two groups. Insulin coma is now seldom used as a treatment for schizophrenia.

Lobotomy

Lobotomy was another popular treatment for this disease. Before the introduction, within the last few years, of the new biology, it was generally believed that human behavior differed from animal behavior because it was controlled by conscience. This specifically human conscience was thought to reside in the prefrontal lobes of the brain. Psychiatrists believed that schizophrenia was a disease of conflict; an overweening conscience was interfering with normal and happy behavior. They therefore sought to do away with the schizophrenic's tyrannical conscience. They simply chopped it off.

In 1936, Antonio Egas Moniz published his famous monograph on the severance of the prefrontal lobes from the rest of the brain. By the mid-'40s, this treatment for schizophrenia was in full swing. In 1949, Egas Moniz received a Nobel Prize for his work on prefrontal lobotomy. About 10,000 patients had been lobotomized in England, and about 25,000 in North America.

By 1951, some doctors were doubting the value of lobotomy. No controlled studies had been done; it was considered unethical to withhold such an obviously useful treatment from patients with so serious a disease as schizophrenia. Gradually, however, the treatment became less popular.

In 1958, Dr. A. A. Robin published a retrospective study of lobotomy in schizophrenia. He found lobotomized patients had not been helped. On the contrary, they remained hospitalized longer than untreated patients. Scarring of the brain produces epilepsy; and 18 percent of the lobotomy patients in this study subsequently developed epilepsy as well as remaining schizophrenic.

Convulsion Therapy

The treatment of schizophrenia by convulsion was introduced to medicine in 1934 by a Hungarian psychiatrist on the strength of a supposed antagonism between epilepsy and schizophrenia. It was later found that the incidence of epilepsy is, in fact, higher in people with schizophrenia than in normal people. The rationale for the treatment has gone, but convulsion therapy remains.

The convulsion is now induced by passing an electric current through the brain. Few proper control studies have been done. It is difficult to disentangle from all the claims and counterclaims whether this treatment is useful or not. In many ways the treatment is like giving a malfunctioning television set a good kick. Rough treatment for a delicate mechanism, the jolt sometimes gets things going again. Convulsion therapy shares with other treatments the advantage that in a desperate situation it at least provides something to do.

Phenothiazine Therapy

Phenothiazines are now the fashionable treatment for schizophrenia. Phenothiazine itself, being toxic to caterpillars, was first used as an insecticide. Veterinary surgeons then found they could use it to deworm animals. A small addition to its chemical structure produced a group of drugs known as the phenothiazines. These were first used in human medicine to prevent shivering during hypothermic or body-cooling surgery. In 1952, two French psychiatrists administered chlorpromazine, one of the first of these new phenothiazine drugs, to agitated psychotic patients, and they noted its extraordinary tranquilizing effect. So started the multimillion dollar business in this major tranquilizer. Within 15 years, chlorpromazine alone had been administered to over 50 million people throughout the world.

The major tranquilizers will quiet wild animals and make them easier to handle. Similarly, these drugs will quiet a patient who is acutely hallucinated, frightened, and disturbed. They will blanket strong feelings. Angry men are made less angry, excited men less excited, and happy men less happy. These drugs are, therefore, useful in the symptomatic treatment of schizophrenia. But just as they are unlikely to cure a tiger of being a tiger, so they are unlikely to cure a schizophrenic of his schizophrenia. The drugs, however, render the patient more approachable.

Many psychiatrists are not convinced of this appraisal of the limited effectiveness of these drugs, which they claim can actually cure schizophrenia. Some psychiatrists feel moral obligation to prescribe these tranquilizers, irrespective of whether the patient is helped by them or not. Some psychiatrists see schizophrenia lurking in the minds of their patients rather as medieval clerics saw the devil hovering alongside the souls of their parishioners. It is these psychiatrists who like to protect the vulnerable among their patients by giving drugs. Holy water was certainly safer and much cheaper.

Megavitamin Therapy

In the early 1950s, a Canadian psychiatrist, Dr. Abram Hoffer, suggested that large, or *mega* doses of vitamin B_3 might prevent the formation in the body of a chemical which he considered to be the cause of schizophrenia. He administered vast doses of this vitamin to schizophrenics, and as is the case with most new treatments, he found that it worked. Dr. Hoffer and his disciples make dramatic claims for the effectiveness of this vitamin.

Recent carefully performed studies into the efficacy of this treatment in schizophrenia have not only failed to confirm that it is useful, but even show that it may have harmful effects. As an explanation of these harmful effects, it has been suggested that the giving of such large doses of one vitamin unbalances the body's normal chemical processes.

A half-century of intensive advertising by the pharmaceutical industry, and the more recent emergence of Adelle Davis and the nutritionists with their praises for health foods, have primed all of us to regard vitamin preparations as essential for our health. Megaton bombs are the most "effective" in our arsenals. To some of us, the therapeutic potential of megavitamins has proved irresistible. Governments are berated because their mental hospitals do not use the megavitamin treatment, and psychiatrists receive angry telephone calls from the relatives of patients who are being deprived of it.

Practically every schizophrenic in the Western world now receives some form of chemotherapy. Those patients who can persuade their psychiatrists to prescribe megavitamins, take them; those patients who can be persuaded by their psychiatrists to accept phenothiazines, take them.

Phenothiazines can suppress some of the symptoms of schizophrenia, and they provide a chemical straitjacket which may diminish difficult behavior. But this straitjacket may also hamper the patient's activities toward recovery. Certainly there are some schizophrenic patients who, with the help of these drugs, manage to lead reasonably normal lives. But there are also other schizophrenic patients who are held by these drugs in a state of apathy, and they cannot lead normal lives again until they are taken off phenothiazines.

No Cheating

Proper drug trials today are "double blind." Half of a group of patients are treated with the drug, and the other half of the patients are treated with an inert substance. Neither the patients nor the doctors know which patients are receiving the drug. Only after all the patients have been assessed for improvement is it revealed which ones have been given the medication.

We have seen that a third of all patients obligingly claim improvement, even when they are given only powdered chalk. The double-blind procedure equalizes the placebo response. Doctors as well as their patients can be drug enthusiasts, and be biased when making an assessment of recovery by actually knowing that a certain patient has received a favorite treatment. The more blind the drug trial, the less useful a drug is generally found to be. Double-blind trials eliminate therapeutic optimism.

Long-term double-blind studies are difficult. Psychiatrists continue to argue about the long-term usefulness of the major tranquilizers. If a patient who is taking such drugs recovers, the question remains whether he would have recovered without them.

Two psychiatrists from Littlemore Hospital, Oxford, published in the *British Journal of Psychiatry* a double-blind study on the use of chlorpromazine. This study revealed that chlorpromazine did not make a scrap of difference in the improvement or otherwise of hospitalized chronic schizophrenic patients. Dr. Nathan Klein, a psychiatrist and the number one drug enthusiast in the United States, then wrote to the *British Journal of Psychiatry:*

> *The excellently designed study of Letemendia and Harris which appeared in the journal for September, on the evaluation of chlorpromazine in the untreated chronic schizophrenic patient, constitutes a real triumph of technique over purpose. The small dose used demonstrates conclusively that inadequate treatment will result in inadequate response. The National Institute of Mental Health cooperative study has already demonstrated that doses of 300 mg. a day of chlorpromazine are ineffective, but it is nice to have this confirmed. The NIH found that doses of 500–600 mg. a day contribute a practical working minimum . . .*

Perhaps Dr. Klein is right. But most British psychiatrists have been using the small-dose regime and claiming that they are doing their patients good. But if they are mistaken in thinking so, so too, perhaps, are the psychiatrists who use the higher-dose regimes. The human element enters in again.

It is not possible to do a double-blind study of the recovery of patients being treated with large doses of chlorpromazine because most such patients walk around like zombies. The psychiatrist assessing recovery can tell at once which patients are taking his favorite drug. He is no longer unbiased.

TB and Mental Illness: A Dismal Comparison

Not much is heard today about chest physicians and tuberculosis; but today, it is hardly possible to open a women's magazine and not read something about the triumphs of modern psychiatric treatments. Let us compare the success that the reticent chest physicians have had with tuberculosis over the last 20 years to the success that voluble psychiatrists have had with mental illness.

In these 20 years, admission rates to mental hospitals have gone up. In the United States, they have risen by 50 percent, and in England they have trebled. Though many of these admissions were, in fact, readmissions, in England there were more new admissions to mental hospitals in 1970 than in 1950. In contrast, the number of admissions for tuberculosis has gone down enormously, having dropped by 75 percent in the United States. In England, in 1950, 26,115 patients with TB required institutional care; but by 1970, the number was so small that the Department of Health and Social Security did not even bother to mention that category in its annual report.

Deaths from suicide, which are considered to be the psychiatrist's concern, fell in England from 4,471 in 1950 to 3,939 in 1970; but in the United States, they rose from 17,145 to 22,060.

The chest physicians did much better. Deaths from tuberculosis in England fell from 15,969 in 1950 to 1,840 in

1970; in the United States, from 33,959 to 5,430.

England records the certified cause of incapacity for all workdays lost by males through illness. In 1950, 13,600,000 days were lost through mental illness. With many new psychiatric treatments to keep people mentally well, 20 years later, the number of days lost climbed to 20,250,000. In contrast, workdays lost through tuberculosis fell 500 percent, from 15,410,000 days a year to 3,010,000.

To control tuberculosis, chest physicians have used a mixture of sensible public health measures, preventive medicine, and rational treatments. Psychiatrists have had no such measures at their disposal. Chest physicians have had success; psychiatrists have not.

Psychiatrists have, however, reduced both the number of patients in mental hospitals and the time that they stay there. English psychiatrists have done best. At the beginning of 1950, there were 140,000 patients in English mental hospitals; in 1970, this number was reduced to 103,269. During the same period, United States psychiatrists reduced the number of their psychiatric beds from 620,000 to 570,000. In these 20 years, psychiatrists have become, and probably quite rightly so, much more liberal in returning disturbed and handicapped people to the community. Certainly with improvements in community care, many such patients can be managed quite adequately outside hospitals.

The removal of so many patients from mental hospitals certainly stands to the credit of psychiatrists. Nevertheless, patients with schizophrenia, the most serious of all mental illnesses, still fill 14 percent of all the occupied hospital beds in Great Britain, and about 25 percent of such beds in the U.S.

Psychiatrists, having failed to find a cure for schizophrenia, have been looking round for greener pastures. They are becoming progressively more concerned with the treatment of two even more common conditions of the mind: anxiety and depression.

SOURCES

Ackner, B., Harris, A., and Oldham, A. J.: "Insulin Treatment of Schizophrenia: A Controlled Study." *Lancet,* 1 607 (1957).

Ayd, Frank J.: "Chlorpromazine: Ten Years' Experience." *Journal of the American Medical Association,* 184 51 (1963).

Bourne, H.: "The Insulin Myth." *Lancet,* 2 964 (1953).

Department of Health and Social Security: *Annual Report for the Year 1970.* London: Her Majesty's Stationery Office, 1971.

Drill's Pharmacology in Medicine: Ed. Joseph R. DiPalma. New York: McGraw-Hill, 1960.

Egas Moniz, A. C. de A. F.: *Tentatives operatoires dans le traitement de certaines psychoses.* Paris: Masson, 1936.

Foulds, G. A.: "Clinical Research in Psychiatry." *Journal of Mental Science,* 102 259 (1958).

Fox, B.: "The Investigation of the Effects of Psychiatric Treatment." *Journal of Mental Science,* 107 493 (1961).

Furbush, Edith M.: "General Paralysis in State Hospitals for Mental Disease." *Archives of Neurology and Psychiatry,* 11 215 (1924).

Gibson, J.: "The Insulin Myth." *Lancet,* 2 1094 (1953).

Glick, B. S., and Margolis, R.: "A Study of the Influence of Experimental Design on the Clinical Outcome in Drug Research." *American Journal of Psychiatry,* 118 1087 (1962).

Hale-White, Sir William: *Great Doctors of the 19th Century.* London: Edward Arnold & Co., 1935.

Hollingshead, A. B., and Redlich, F. C.: *Social Class and Mental Illness: A Community Study.* New York: John Wiley & Sons, Inc., 1958.

Javrik, Murray E.: "Drugs Used in the Treatment of Psychiatric Disorders." In *The Pharmacological Basis of Therapeutics.* Ed. Louis S. Goodman and Alfred Gilman, New York: Macmillan Co., 1965.

Kind, Hans: "The Psychogenesis of Schizophrenia: A Review of the Literature." *International Journal of Psychiatry,* 3 383 (1967).

Kline, Nathan S.: "Chlorpromazine in Chronic Schizophrenia." *British Journal of Psychiatry,* 113 950 (1967).

Leighton, A. H.; Hughes, Charles C.; Tremblay, Marc-adelard; Harding, John S.; Rapaport, Robert N.; Macmillan, Allistear; and Leighton, Dorothea C.: *The Stirling County Study of Psychiatric Disorder and Sociocultural Environment.* Vols. I–III. New York: Basic Books, Inc., 1959–63.

Letemendia, F. J. J., and Harris, A. D.: "Chlorpromazine and the Untreated Chronic Schizophrenic." *British Journal of Psychiatry,* 113 950 (1967).

Miller, S. M., and Mishler, E. G.: "Social Class, Mental Illness and American Psychiatry." In *Mental Health of the Poor.* Ed. Frank Riessman, Jerome Cohen, and Arthur Pearl. New York: Free Press, 1964.

Ministry of Health: *Annual Report for the Year 1950.* London: Her Majesty's Stationery Office, 1951.

Registrar General: *Statistical Review of England and Wales for the Year 1950.* London: Her Majesty's Stationery Office, 1951.

————: *Statistical Review of England and Wales for the Year 1970.* London: Her Majesty's Stationery Office, 1971.

Robin, A. A.: "A Retrograde Controlled Study of Leucotomy in Schizophrenia Affective Disorders." *Journal of Mental Science,* 104 1025 (1958).

Shepherd, M., Cooper, B., Brown, A. C., and Kalton, G. W.: *Psychiatric Illness and General Practice.* London: Oxford University Press, 1966.

Siegel, Malcolm, and Tefft, Harold: "'Pink Spot' and Its Components in Normal and Schizophrenic Urine." *Journal of Nervous and Mental Diseases,* 152 412 (1971).

Sim, Myre: *Guide to Psychiatry.* Edinburgh and London: E. N. S. Livingstone Ltd., 1968.

Srole, L., Langner, T. S., Michael, S. T., Opler, M. K., and Rennie, T. A. C.: *Mental Health in the Metropolis: The Midtown Manhattan Study in Social Psychiatry.* Ed. Thomas A. C. Rennie. New York: McGraw-Hill, 1962.

Terman, Lewis: Genetic Studies of Genius. Vol. 4. *The Gifted Child Grows Up*. Stanford: Stanford University Press, 1926–59.

Tooth, G. C., and Newton, M. P.: *Leucotomy in England and Wales 1942–45*. London: Her Majesty's Stationery Office, 1961.

Tyler, L. E.: *The Psychology of Human Differences*. New York: Appleton, 1956.

U. S. Bureau of Census: *Statistical Abstract of the U.S.A.* Washington, D.C.: Government Printing Office, 1971.

Drugs for the Mind

Depression and anxiety are unpleasant. There are few of us who do not quite often experience these twin discomforts of the mind. Indeed, depression and anxiety are so common that they are probably biologically useful.

Hens in a pen soon develop a pecking order. The one at the top eats the best worms, sits where she likes, and pecks all the others. The one at the bottom eats what is left, sits. in a draft, and can peck no one. In her own bird-brained way, she must feel anxious, depressed, and inadequate. This may be uncomfortable for her, but without these feelings, she would peck back and feathers would fly, and she'd come off the worse.

The Uses of Anxiety

Biologists studying animal behavior and human behavior find that dominant-submissive relationships exist in all groups. Such relationships diminish intragroup aggression. It seems probable that for humans, too, feelings of constraint and inadequacy are the normal accompaniment of submissive behavior, and that climbing the dominance ladder provokes anxiety. When anxiety is abolished by drinking, for instance, intragroup fighting and serious injury become more common.

If everyone always felt self-confident, adequate, and energetic, everyone would want to be boss. Social cohesion would no longer be possible, and our very survival would become more doubtful.

Anxiety is an inevitable part of creative concern. It is an

unlucky child whose parents stop worrying about him. "Worry work" or the worrying that many people do about possible future difficulties helps them to cope with such difficulties if and when they actually happen. Happy people are said to worry more than unhappy people; they are making sure that their lives continue to go well.

Accepting Life

Truth is, of course, a malleable commodity, but some truths are reasonably immortal. Probably one of these truths is that we cannot really escape from feelings of depression and anxiety, for such feelings are a part of our very being. An Oriental philosopher, when asked if he could sum up the answer to happiness in one word, answered, "yes." If a man can say yes to the fact that he may get fired from his job, his mistress may take another lover, his wife may divorce him, his children may smoke pot, he may drop dead from a heart attack, or his sister may get raped, then he can be reasonably sure of never needing a psychiatrist—that is, as long as his brain holds out.

The Oriental philosopher was prepared to accept all that life might bring, including unhappiness and worry. Certainly unhappiness and worry are unpleasant, and few of us are foolish enough to want to suffer them unnecessarily. But can we escape them?

"He who would have his life must lose it," it is written in the Bible. Perhaps it is only when we are prepared to face even death that we can start truly living.

Pharmaceutical psychiatry does not encourage such an outlook. It offers escape from anxiety and depression by treatment so that the effort to come to terms with misery, worry, death, and disaster need not be made.

But how successful are such treatments? Within the last few years, many new drugs for the treatment of anxiety and depression have been introduced into clinical medicine and are now widely used. But we do not seem any happier.

Drugs and Suicide

Analysis of the annual suicide rates for England and the United States from the beginning of this century on shows that an economic depression makes us miserable and more of us commit suicide. On the contrary, a good war cheers us up and fewer people do away with themselves. But the introduction of all these new drugs for depression and anxiety does not appear to have had any noticeable effect upon the suicide rate. Actually, since their introduction, our rates of attempted suicide have gone up faster than a guided missle. The most popular poisons used to attempt suicide are the very drugs doctors prescribe to cheer us up and make us stop worrying.

The suicide rate for psychiatrists, who have the easiest access to such drugs, continues to top suicides in all other professions. Doctors tend to use these drugs more than other people. And these drugs do not seem to do *them* much good. This was shown in a 20-year follow-up study of 268 college students from Massachusetts, 45 of whom had become physicians. These physicians used amphetamines twice as often, and sedatives three to four times as often, as did those in the non-medical group. Eventually, three of the 45 physicians were hospitalized for overusage of drugs.

Five groups of drugs are commonly used to alter one's state of mind: major tranquilizers, opiates, hallucinogens, anti-anxiety drugs, and anti-depressants and stimulants.

Major Tranquilizers

The major tranquilizers include the phenothiazines which are used for the treatment of schizophrenia. But the manufacturers of these particular drugs suggest that their use should not be confined to schizophrenics. Drug literature works to persuade doctors that these drugs are also useful for problems as varied as rebellious toddlers, delinquent teenagers, and anxious adults.

Phenothiazines can be dangerous. Jaundice, impotence,

skin rashes, and an often fatal blood disorder are a few of the long list of disorders that they can cause.

Though nobody knows how they work, phenothiazines are the most frequently used major tranquilizers. They interfere with such an array of the body's chemical processes that it is not yet possible to say exactly how these drugs produce their clinical effects, nor indeed how harmful they can be. Laboratory studies made on rats treated with chlorpromazine for various periods of time and in dosages equivalent to those used in man showed that some of these rats developed irreversible brain damage.

After many years on phenothiazines, some patients develop continual grimacing and writhing movements of their mouth, jaw, and tongue. Phenothiazines may or may not be able to cure madness, but they have certainly made people look crazy. And this effect is permanent. The drug can be stopped, but the grimaces continue.

Opiates

Opiates are the oldest of all the tranquilizers. Opium comes from the opium poppy, and morphine is its purified product. These drugs were used extensively in the past as tranquilizers, hypnotics, and pain relievers. "Of all the remedies which it has pleased Almighty God to give to man to relieve his suffering, none is so universal and so efficacious as opium," wrote Thomas Sydenham, a 17th-century physician and a father of English medicine. For a man in severe pain, opium was and is a miraculous drug. But opium, like all other successful treatments, is misused, and patients get hooked on it.

Enlightened doctors were soon complaining of opium's misuse. In 18th-century England, Dr. George Young wrote that opium had "got into the hands of every pretender of practice, and is prescribed every day not only by many charitable and well-meaning ladies, but even by the too officious and ignorant nurses." He complained that "great numbers are daily destroyed; not, indeed, by such doses as kill suddenly

---

OPIUM and **Morphine Habit Cured** in **10** to **80** days. Refer to 1000 patients cured in all parts. **Dr. Marsh, Quincy, Mich.**

In the latter years of the 19th century, opiate addiction became a grave problem on both sides of the Atlantic. Many people became hooked on opium or morphine by taking patent medicines for minor ills. Drs. Marsh and Carlton evidently believed that what patent medicines could cause, patent medicines could cure.

OPIUM and **Morphine habit cured painless: No Publicity. Dr. CARLTON,** 187 Washington St., Chicago, Ill.

. . . but by its being given unseasonably in such diseases and to such constitutions for which it is not proper." He considered its use in "hysterics and nervous disorders" as on a par with giving "pills to purge folly."

Doctors prescribed opium freely, and many patent medicines contained opium. Consequently, opium addiction became a serious problem throughout Europe and America. In 1884, the then superintendent of the Toronto asylum in which I work complained in the *Toronto Daily Globe* of the increasing numbers of opium addicts being admitted to his hospital.

The opium habit is a terrible vice, and so rapidly spreading that many doctors will not tell their patients what medication they are taking, when they administer it. It is prescribed for nervousness and insomnia and the patient is tempted to continue the use of the drug, even after the occasion for its use is past.

Having gotten their patients addicted to opium, doctors looked around for other drugs with which to cure them. In 1885, two doctors from the German Morphine Institute confirmed the value of cocaine, which was said to be free from addictive properties.

In 1898, Heinrich Dresser in Germany altered the chemical structure of morphine to produce heroin. Heroin was claimed to have all the therapeutic advantages of opium, but to be free from all addictive properties; it was especially recommended in the treatment of opium addiction. Seldom had a new remedy been heralded with so much enthusiasm. Opium addicts were also enthusiastic. They took the heroin and found that they preferred it.

Methadone (Physeptone) is a synthetic pain-killer that was first produced in Germany and introduced into clinical medicine at the end of World War II. In 1964, the first methadone center for heroin addicts was established in New York. Heroin addicts are weaned off their heroin and maintained on regular doses of methadone. Impressive results have been claimed for its use; but after six years of experience, some doctors are questioning the value of methadone.

Today, methadone is being "pushed" on the streets. It does indeed make a very adequate substitute for heroin.

A medley of morphine, cocaine, heroin, and methadone is easily available to anyone who wishes to try them. It is estimated that in the United States alone, 55,000 people were addicted to the opiates in 1960, and 500,000—nearly 10 times as many—in 1972. For centuries opium was the doctors' favorite drug. Time has not lessened its kick.

Hallucinogens

Hallucinogens are used by the more adventurous to explore different states of mind, and this sometimes may be useful. The hallucinogens are not physically addictive, though they are used by some as a convenient way to opt out permanently from this world.

The hallucinogenic drugs are not accepted as treatment, and therefore serious side effects were soon found for them. A state commissioner for the blind erroneously announced that six Pennsylvania students on LSD had been blinded while staring into the sun. Newspapers announced the commissioner's finding with large headlines and retracted it a few days later with small ones.

LSD was reported to cause chromosomal bruising, and has been publicized as a cause of malformed babies. When it was learned that some of our favorite treatment drugs, including barbiturates and aspirin, may also cause chromosomal bruising, the subject was quickly forgotten.

Like all biologically active drugs, hallucinogens may indeed have untoward and unexpected side effects, but it is difficult to evaluate their seriousness. The hallucinogens and the Pill are the shady drugs of our society; their side effects are overreported almost to the extent that the side effects of our treatment drugs are underreported.

Anti-Anxiety Drugs

The anti-worry drugs are the most popular and widely used of all the drugs for the mind. The names of many of them are now household words: alcohol, chloral, paraldehyde, glutethamide (Doriden), meprobamate (Equanil and Miltown), chlordiazepexide (Librium), diazepam (Valium), barbiturates (Sodium Amytal, Seconal, Soneryl, and Nembutal).

The pharmacologist knows these drugs as central nervous system depressants. The central nervous system consists of the brain and spinal cord. These drugs are brain poisons. They are called depressants because they depress the brain function, not because they make people feel depressed. In fact, when first used, they usually make people feel less so.

The use of alcohol, one of man's most popular treatments, extends back into prehistory. In the last century alcohol was used as a treatment for insanity. A hundred years ago, the expenditure on beer, spirits, and wines at the Toronto mental hospital with which I am associated far exceeded the money spent on other drugs and medicines. In 1877, a report that criticized alcohol as a treatment for insanity was vigorously refuted by the hospital superintendent as "a sweeping indictment . . . against the medical treatment of nearly all the asylums of Europe and America."

Alcohol is now seldom used as a treatment for the insane. However, a recent report showed that a group of old men attending a psychiatric rehabilitation clinic were treated with beer and did better than another group dosed with Largactil. Largactil is the current fashionable drug for the treatment of lunacy. Beer is cheaper, and the patients like it more.

In France, which has the world's highest per capita consumption of alcohol, 10 percent of all deaths are due to cirrhosis of the liver or to other diseases directly attributable to alcohol. Many additional deaths due to infections and accidents are also indirectly attributable to this drug. Perhaps French wines are delectable enough to make an early death acceptable, but it is difficult to convincingly argue that alcohol is good for health. Nevertheless, the answers to a questionnaire showed that four-fifths of the French thought wine good for the health, and a fourth held that it was indispensable. People are always prepared to overlook the disadvantages of their favorite treatments.

The use of chloral and paraldehyde goes back to the last century. Barbiturates were introduced into clinical medicine in 1903, and were used in ever increasing amounts until the last few years. They have been partly supplanted by the newer and more expensive depressants: Doriden, Equanil, Librium, Valium, and many others. Small amounts of these drugs bring release from anxiety; large amounts bring death. Sleep and coma are stages in between.

All depressants impair judgment and slow down reactions. A group of 68 drivers who were taking one of the newer of these drugs had six major and 10 minor car accidents in 90 days. This is a tenfold increase in the normally predicted accident rate.

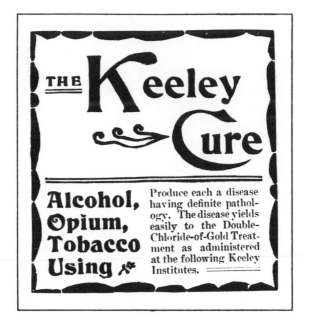

THE **K**eeley **C**ure

Alcohol, Opium, Tobacco Using Produce each a disease having definite pathology. The disease yields easily to the Double-Chloride-of-Gold Treatment as administered at the following Keeley Institutes.

Dr. Keeley's Institutes advertised that they had returned a third of a million inebriated Americans to sobriety with their bichloride-of-gold cure. Gold may cure an itching palm, but it is doubtful that its salts ever cured an alcoholic. Today drugs like Librium are alleged by their manufacturers to help alcoholics stop drinking. Many alcoholics, however, get intoxicated on Librium instead, or mix it with alcohol to reduce the cost of getting drunk.

Barbiturates are addictive; habitual users become tense and anxious. The cause of this increasing anxiety is often not recognized. Dr. William Sargeant reports having seen several anxious patients who were lobotomized because of their crippling anxiety. Only later was it determined that their anxiety was caused by barbiturate intoxication.

Chronic intoxication with barbiturates causes personality deterioration. Like the alcoholic, the barbiturate addict loses his job, his family, and his friends. He becomes maudlin, moody, and childish. At the Federal treatment center for drug addiction at Lexington, Kentucky, it has been found that addiction to the barbiturates causes greater physical and personality deterioration than does addiction to opiates. The

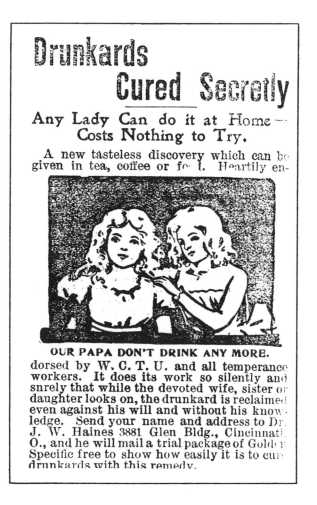

Drunkards
Cured Secretly

Any Lady Can do it at Home — Costs Nothing to Try.

A new tasteless discovery which can be given in tea, coffee or fo· i. Heartily en-

OUR PAPA DON'T DRINK ANY MORE.

dorsed by W. C. T. U. and all temperance workers. It does its work so silently and snrely that while the devoted wife, sister or daughter looks on, the drunkard is reclaimed even against his will and without his knowledge. Send your name and address to Dr. J. W. Haines 3881 Glen Bldg., Cincinnati, O., and he will mail a trial package of Golden Specific free to show how easily it is to cure drunkards with this remedy.

Drunkards may have been treated discreetly with Dr. Haines' remedy, but they were not treated effectively.

barbiturate addict takes frequent overdoses; he makes constant work for hospitals.

The chronic anxiety of a regular user of barbiturates is made worse when he stops using the drug. Then withdrawal insomnia adds to his discomfort. This increased anxiety and insomnia makes him reluctant to relinquish his drug. Like the alcoholic, the barbiturate user whose drugs are cut off may suffer DT's (delirium tremens) and withdrawal epileptic fits.

The Chinese who said, "I no drinkee for drinkee; I drinkee for drunkee" was probably in trouble. Most people realize that it is all right to drink for fun, but not to drink to escape one's problems. The problems go on, and so does the drinking. Similarly, it may be all right to take mood-altering drugs for fun, but it is unwise to take them for the reason that otherwise life would be too uncomfortable. Yet doctors offer barbiturates to those very people who are seeking to avoid their troubles. When the drugs work, their patients are in deeper trouble: they cannot manage with them, and they cannot manage without them.

Barbiturates can be obtained legally only through a doctor. In the United States, 250 tons of them are sold each year. With such truckloads of them around, one can be sure the people have had their fair share of trouble with them. So have the British. In Great Britain, half a million people are regular users of barbiturates; 110,000 are firmly hooked on them.

Doctors are the most successful of all drug peddlers. Only a few heroin pushers in the world's great cities have been anywhere near so successful.

Jacqueline Susann, in her best selling novel *The Valley of the Dolls*, gives a dramatic account of an actress' addiction to barbiturates, her degradation and death. The lay public knows the dangers of barbiturates; the medical profession does not seem so well informed. In 1954, a *Lancet* editorial said that barbiturates are "true drugs of addiction," causing a risk that is "the least appreciated and the most sinister." However, the editorial saw "evidence that the high noon of their popularity is passing." *Lancet* was wrong.

Prescriptions for barbiturates in England doubled between 1953 and 1959. By the early 1960s, the increase in their use started to level off, but only because barbiturates were being replaced by the newer and more expensive central nervous system depressants. Drug manufacturers claimed innocence for each of these new drugs.

Expensive meprobamate was the first of these new drugs. In 1955, it was marketed in the United States as Miltown; in Britain, as Equanil. Its manufacturers popularized it by laying great stress upon its safety. In the United States, meprobamate was a great money spinner, but many millions of dollars, 14 billion tablets and 500 million doctors' prescriptions later, it became apparent that the undesirable effects of Miltown differed little from those of the barbiturates.

The other non-barbiturate depressants are all also several times more expensive than barbiturates. Each in its turn has been shown to cause states of intoxication and physical dependence clinically similar to those induced by barbiturates.

Anxiety is unpleasant; nobody likes it. The more effective a drug is at relieving it, the more it will be a drug of addiction. There can only be one safe drug for the treatment of anxiety: a drug that does not work. A brain chronically intoxicated with depressant drugs does not function well. By giving such drugs to patients who are already having difficulties in managing their lives, doctors add to their patients' problems.

Stimulants and Anti-Depressants

Stimulants and anti-depressants are prescribed to give people more energy and to cheer them up. The stimulants include: the amphetamines, dextroamphetamine (Dexedrine), and methylamphetamine (Methadrine, "speed"), methylphenidate (Ritalin), and phenmetrizine (Preludin). In the group of anti-depressants are imipramine (Totranil), amitriptyline (Elavil), and many others besides.

Amphetamines were introduced into medicine in 1936; and since then, they have been causing increasing trouble. Because they elevate the mind and depress the appetite, they are used for the treatment of both depression and obesity. But their use in depression is followed by rebound fatigue and more depression, and the user is left feeling more miserable than before.

Nor are the amphetamines any more useful for obesity. Tolerance is soon developed to their appetite-suppressant effect. The obese, being on the whole more lazy than the rest of us, like to rely on drugs to make them thin, rather than upon themselves to make the effort to eat less.

Once experienced, the exhilaration produced by amphetamines is difficult to resist. Fat people are demonstrations of the inability to cope with the temptation to overeat; it is hardly surprising, then, that they cannot resist amphetamines.

In 1966, British National Health Service general practitioners prescribed 200 million tablets of amphetamines or related substances, mostly to middle-aged housewives. Coincidentally, the most frequent forgeries of National Health Service prescriptions were being made by women between the ages of 30 and 50, and were for amphetamines.

The young learn best from example. Teenagers have now taken up their mothers' habits.

Speed Kills

The craze for intravenous amphetamine was nurtured in California. By 1962, half a million ampuls of methadrine were being distributed to drugstores in the San Francisco area. At the request of the Attorney General of California, drug companies stopped supplying the drug to the local pharmacies. But this did not stop the use of intravenous amphetamine; the amphetamine user soon found alternative sources of supply. Amphetamines are easy to concoct, and any intelligent chemistry student can make them at home.

Several countries are introducing legislation to control amphetamines; but now that the medical profession and pharmaceutical companies have established their use, these drugs are probably here to stay.

Intravenous amphetamines came to Great Britain when the Dangerous Drugs Regulations of 1968 removed from all doctors, except those working in special treatment centers, the right to prescribe heroin and cocaine to addicts. Some doctors—either because they were "too kind" to resist their patients' pleas for drugs, or for personal gain—prescribed methylamphetamine instead. The new craze for intravenous amphetamines soon caught on. By the summer of 1968, it had resulted in an epidemic in London of "meth heads" and "speed freaks."

The effects of intravenous amphetamines are considerably more disastrous than those of heroin and cocaine. Many young people now become psychotic through methadrine misuse. "Speed kills."

The Japanese Connection

Western countries were not, in fact, the first to get hooked on amphetamines. They became popular in Japan during World War II, and their popularity has continued. By 1954, between 200,000 and 1 million Japanese, mostly between the ages of 16 and 25, were estimated to be addicted to amphetamines. Chronic amphetamine intoxication causes madness and permanent brain damage. It also produces in the user a dangerous combination of a suspicious mood and violent behavior. Amphetamine misuse was involved in half of 60 murder cases that occurred in one large Japanese city during May and June, 1954.

In 1954, the Japanese Government introduced strict controls on the manufacture and use of amphetamines. In the same year, the Chief Medical Officer of Britain's Ministry of Health wrote of amphetamines in his annual Report:

The drugs of this group have the advantage of being relatively non-toxic; addiction to them is rare, and there are no serious ill effects.

Almost certainly, this was no sinister plot by the Ministry of Health to make all the English sick and thereby increase the importance of the ministry; they probably did not know what was happening in Japan. But drug manufacturers collect extensive information about their products. Is it possible that the manufacturers of amphetamines were also unaware of the dangers of these drugs? Amphetamines were selling well.

The Cheery Cure

Isoniazid is widely used in the treatment of tuberculosis. People with T.B. have their fair share of troubles. As an unexpected side effect of isoniazid, it was found that it cheered them up. Thus, in the early 1950s, the first of the anti-depressants came into clinical use. So started yet another multimillion dollar business and a drug company race to bring out new and "better" anti-depressants, most of which vary only in their cost and capsule color.

Now widely used in the treatment of depression, anti-depressants probably work in a way similar to amphetamines, though their pharmacological action is slower and generally less dramatic. Some studies show that anti-depressants make people feel better while other studies show that they are no more useful than placebos. The fact that some users are addicted to them is strong supporting evidence that they can be mood elevators. A kickback depression may be expected to follow their use.

A speaker at the 1969 symposium of the World Psychiatric Association noted that depression appeared to be becoming more common in Europe. He said he was seeing patients who no longer had symptom-free periods between their acute episodes of depression. He suggested that the use of the anti-depressants was making depression a more chronic disease.

The Pot and Kettle Story

Reducing pills, the anti-depressant group of drugs, and the barbiturates are regarded by the Establishment as the "nice" drugs because they are used by the respectable middle-aged. The fact that drug abuse is more common in the middle-aged than in the younger generation may not be obvious from perusal of the daily papers. But then teenagers do not write for the press. Let Lenny Bruce speak for the hippie generation.

FIRST WOMAN

To serve on a jury in a civil case is easy, but when you're dealing with drug addicts it's rough. This damned jury duty has me a nervous wreck. I had to take five sleeping pills to get some rest last night. You build up a tolerance to the damned things so quickly. I feel miserable today. I'm really dragging.

SECOND WOMAN

Here, take one of these dexies.

FIRST WOMAN

What are they for?

SECOND WOMAN

They're amphetamine, Dexedrine spansules. My doctor gave them to me for depression and fatigue. They really give you a lift. I take them all the time except when it's "that time of the month"—then I take Demerol.

THIRD WOMAN

(Rummaging through her purse and producing a handful of pills.) Do you know what these red and white ones are? My neighbor's doctor gave them to her to try out. They're supposed to be for nerves. Better than Miltowns.

SECOND WOMAN

Oh, those are Deprols. Umm, no, wait a minute, I think they're phenobarbs.
(An elderly woman juror, silent until now, turns and speaks)

Drug abuse is often just what the doctor unwittingly ordered. For the most part, doctors are men of average good will, and probably only a very few prescribe harmful drugs malevolently. Doctors are trained to be helpful, to make people feel better. Most people will not refuse their boozing friend a drink, even though they know the drink isn't good for him; and most doctors will not refuse a patient a drug if he insists he is too unhappy to manage without it.

It is, of course, no easy matter to decide if an individual has the right to take a potentially harmful substance. A doctor's duty is much more straightforward. From the time of Hippocrates, doctors have accepted as part of their professional code that they shall do no harm. Doctors are now prescribing dangerous drugs, and they are doing this unwisely.

In 1968, the British Medical Association Council appointed a working committee to inquire into the medical uses of amphetamines. It concluded that amphetamines have only a very small part to play in legitimate medical practice and they recommended means by which the medical profession could control their use. By the next year, the improper prescription of amphetamines had reached such proportions that the Society of Pharmacists advised its members not to honor prescriptions for injectable amphetamines.

Frank W. Horner Limited recommends its drug Solacen for the intelligent young mother who cannot settle into happy domesticity. This advertisement was last used in 1967; it no longer conforms to the pharmaceutical firm's advertising policy.

When constant worry begins to oppress...

Solacen
lightens the load of worry

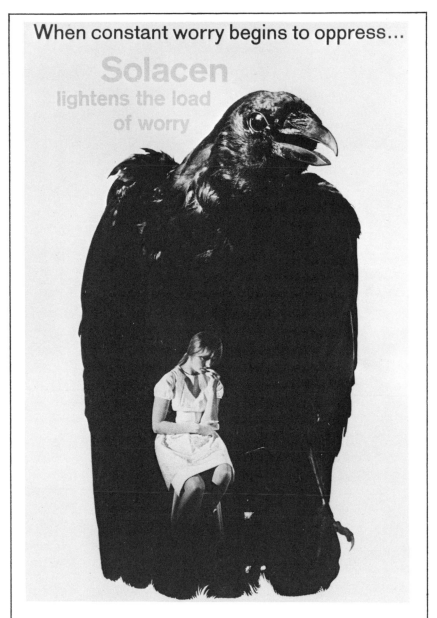

for the anxious housewife

College seems like yesterday. Suddenly the excitement of a vital social and business world seems buried forever.

She welcomed marriage, children, domesticity. But sometimes the change seems too much, too sudden. She is frustrated and lonely.

To lighten her load of worry comes new Solacen. Solacen—a new tranquilizer with a wider range of neurotic symptom improvement.

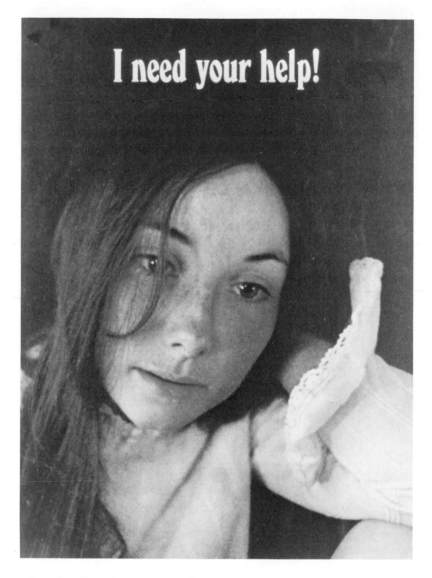

I need your help!

Smith, Kline & French Laboratories suggest the use of chlorpromazine, a major tranquilizer, for this girl. Their advertisement states: "Whether it's expressed verbally or implied through actions or complaints, many patients need help in coping with overwhelming anxiety. . . . Let's give them the help they need."

The medical profession has always had difficulty in policing itself; doctors like their professional freedom. Forming rules for their ordinary affairs is difficult; but forming rules for the hallowed realm of treatment is almost impossible. Every doctor fights for the right to decide for himself his patient's treatment, and his patients want him to have that right. Medicine expands its frontiers, and doctors make themselves responsible for the alleviation of our mental discomforts. The drugs that do this the best are, of course, the ones we like the best. They are the drugs of addiction.

The Giant Drug Pushers

Not only patients encourage doctors to prescribe addictive drugs, but so do the drug companies. Drug companies exist to make money. Drugs for the mind are now the big money makers, and drug companies use every means—from salesmen to copious advertisements in medical journals to direct mail advertising—to encourage every doctor to prescribe their products. One English general practitioner estimated that he was receiving 14 pounds of advertising mail a month.

English drug firms spend $36 million a year advertising their products to doctors. I have not been able to find out how much the American drug companies spend, since this information is not readily available. One author quotes this figure as $750 million. There are about 330,000 doctors in the United States, and if this figure of $750 million is correct, then each doctor gets about $2,250 spent on him each year to encourage him to prescribe drugs. Throughout his professional career, this certainly adds up to considerably more money than is spent on his medical education. Like everybody else, doctors respond to advertising campaigns. Perhaps it is not surprising that doctors prescribe dangerous drugs unwisely.

I wished to show some examples of the many hundreds of advertisements put out by drug companies which suggest to doctors the use of drugs for all sorts of everyday situations. I am grateful to the few companies that granted me permission to reproduce their advertisements. CIBA Pharmaceutical Company would not permit me to use their ad showing a man with a megaphone head. Doctors were urged to use CIBA's Ritalin (a habit-forming drug, by the way) for "environmental depression" caused by "NOISE: a new social problem." Merck, Sharp

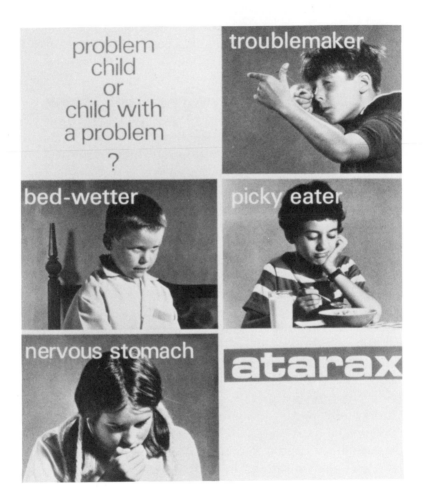

Pfizer recommends its anti-anxiety drug Atarax to treat children.

and Dohme pictures a heavily made-up woman with "Lady, your anxiety is showing" written across her face. Triavil, their mixture of an anti-depressant and a major tranquilizer, would deal with both her depression and anxiety.

U.S.V. Pharmaceutical Corporation's gorgeous young woman with a "swimsuit by Jantzen and a body by Dexaspan" pushed their strongly habit-forming mixture of amphetamine and barbiturate. Geigy Corporation shows a man with a hundred-pound weight for a head. He should be given their anti-depressant Tofranil, "when depression comes to mind."

Ads Sandoz Pharmaceuticals would not allow to be shown suggest the use of their major tranquilizer, Mellaril, for the doctor's "little patient," "Dennis the Menace," with whom "a quiet moment is unknown," "and here's Sulky Sue, what shall we do".

Neither could I show Eli Lilly and Company's ad which recommends their anti-depressant Aventyl for the man who "tries to hide fear behind bravado." Nor a picture of their Tuinal Capsule, an expensive mixture of barbiturates, which wishes you "good night."

Pharmaceutical companies continually bring out new drugs for the mind, and the evidence is fairly clear that their ever wider use will create yet more trouble for the future. Until doctors and their patients get together to work out such guidelines, the medical profession will remain society's number one drug peddler of dangerous drugs, and society will continue to have a problem foisted upon it each time a drug company brings out yet another mood-altering drug. Often the state or insurance companies pay for an individual's use of these drugs; pot smokers and drinkers at least pay for their own.

SOURCES

Ambrose, Myles, Director, Drug Abuse Law Enforcement, Dept. of Justice, as reported by UPI (Washington), Jan. 29, 1972.

Arnold, O. H.: Report in "The Uses and Abuses of Psychiatry." Symposium World Psychiatric Association. *Documenta Geigy,* Geigy Pharmaceuticals, Nov. 1969.

Bastide, M.: "Une enquête sur l'opinion publique à l'égard de *l'alcoolisme." Population,* **9** 13 (1954).

Bosworth, David M.: "Iproniazid: A Brief Review of Its Introduction and Clinical Use." *Annals of the New York Academy of Sciences,* **80** (Art 3) 809 (1959).

Bowles, Grover G.: "New Treatment for Addicts: New Control Problem for Pharmacists." *Modern Hospital,* **114** 126 (1970).

Brandon, S., and Smith, D.: "Amphetamines in General Practice." *Journal of the College of General Practitioners,* **5** 603 (1961).

British Medical Association Council: Annual Report. *British Medical Journal Supplement,* **2** 71 (1968).

British Medical Journal: "Voluntary Restriction of Amphetamines." **4** 532 (1968).

Bruce, Lenny: "How to Talk Dirty and Influence People." *Playboy,* Nov. 1963.

Ching-piao Chien: In Report from A.P.A. meeting at San Francisco. *Geriatric Focus,* **9** (8) 5 (1970).

Clark, Daniel: "Insanity's Borderland": *Daily Globe* (Toronto), Nov. 29, 1884.

————: *Report of the Medical Superintendent of the Asylum for the Insane, Toronto, for the Year Ending September 30, 1878.*

Connell, Philip H.: "Clinical Manifestations and Treatment of Amphetamine Type of Dependence." *Journal of the American Medical Association,* **196** 718 (1966).

Council of Society of Pharmacists of Great Britain: "Statement on Amphetamine Sulphate Powder." *Pharmaceutical Journal,* **202** 257 (1969).

Denber, Herman C. B.: "Tranquilizers in Psychiatry." In Freedman and Kaplan, *Comprehensive Textbook of Psychiatry.* Baltimore: Williams and Wilkins Co., 1967.

Dishotsky, Norman I., Loughman, Wm. D., Mogar, Robert E., and Lipscomb, Wendell R.: "LSD and Genetic Damage." *Science,* **172** 431 (1971).

Editorial Archives of Environmental Health: "Heroin Addiction. The Epidemic of the 70's." **21** 589 (1970).

Essig, C. F.: "Addiction to Non-Barbiturate Sedatives and Tranquilizing Drugs." *Clinical Pharmacology and Therapeutics,* **5** 334 (1964).

Glatt, M. M.: "The Abuse of Barbiturates in the United Kingdom." *Bulletin on Narcotics,* **14** 19 (1962).

Hawks, D., Mitcheson, M., Ogborne, A., and Edwards, Griffith: "Abuse of Methylamphetamines." *British Medical Journal,* **2** 715 (1969).

Hunter, R. A., Earl, C. J., and Thornicroft, S.: "An Apparently Irreversible Syndrome of Abnormal Movements Following Phenothiazine Medication." *Proceedings of the Royal Society of Medicine,* **57** 758 (1964).

Hunter, Richard, and MacAlpine, Ida: *Three Hundred Years of Psychiatry. 1535–1860.* London: Oxford University Press, 1963.

Isbell, Harris: "Manifestations and Treatment of Addiction to Narcotic Drugs and Barbiturates." *Medical Clinics of North America,* **34** 425 (1950).

Javrik, Murray E.: "Drugs Used in the Treatment of Psychiatric Disorders." In *The Pharmacological Basis of Therapeutics.* Ed. Louis S. Goodman and Alfred Gilman. New York: Macmillan Co., 1965.

Katz, Sidney: "Doctors Warned About Deadly 'Cure' for Heroin Addiction." *Toronto Daily Star,* Oct. 10, 1970.

Klerman, G. L., and Cole, J. O.: "Clinical Pharmacology of Imipramine and Related Antidepressant Compounds." *Pharmacology Reviews,* **17** 101 (1965).

Lancet: "Shadow Over the Barbiturates." **2** 75 (1954).

Lemere, Frederick: "The Danger of Amphetamine Dependency." *American Journal of Psychiatry,* **123** 569 (1966).

Leyburn, Peter: "A Critical Look at Antidepressant Trials." *Lancet,* 2 1135.

Ministry of Health: *Annual Report for the Year 1954.* London: Her Majesty's Stationery Office, 1955.

——: *Report of the Interdepartmental Committee. Drug Addiction.* London: Her Majesty's Stationery Office, 1961.

Modell, W.: "Status and Prospect of Drugs for Overeating: Report to the Council on Drugs of the A.M.A." *Journal of the American Medical Association,* **173** 1131 (1960).

Nagahama, M.: "A Review of Drug Abuse and Counter Measures in Japan Since World War II." *Bulletin on Narcotics,* **20** (3) 19 (1968).

Quirano, Jean-Pierre: "La consommation d'alcool en France." *L'information médicale et paramédicale,* Feb. 3, 1970.

Rogers, J. Maurice: "Drug Abuse—Just What the Doctor Ordered." *Psychology Today,* Sept. 1971.

Russo, J. Robert: *Amphetamine Abuse.* Springfield, Ill.: Charles C. Thomas, 1968.

Sargent, Wm.: "Discussion on Sedation and Stimulation of Man." *Proceedings of the Royal Society of Medicine,* **51** 353 (1958).

Shatan, Chaim: "Withdrawal Symptoms After Abrupt Termination of Imipramine." *Journal of the Canadian Psychiatric Association,* 2 S151 (1966).

Smidt, H., and Rank, C.: *In Berliner Klinische Wochenschrift,* Sept. 14, 1885. Quoted in: *Abstracts and Extracts. American Journal of Insanity,* Jan. 1886.

Sommer, H., and Quandt, J.: "Langzeitbehandlung mit Chlorpromazine im Tierexperiment." *Fortschritte Der Neurologie, Psychiatrie und Ihrer Grenzgebiete,* **38** 466 (1970).

Susann, Jacqueline: *Valley of the Dolls.* New York: Bantam Books, 1970.

Terry, C. E., and Pellens, M.: *The Opium Problem.* New York: Bureau of Social Hygiene Inc., 1928.

The Times (London): "Students on L.S.D. Blinded by Sun." Jan. 15 and Jan. 19, 1968.

Vaillant, G. E., Brighton, J. R., and McArthur, C.: "Physicians' Use of Mood Altering Drugs." *New England Journal of Medicine,* **282** 365 (1970).

Walsh, John: "Methadone and Heroin Addiction: Without a Cure." *Science,* **168** (1970).

Wilson, Allen T., and Hooper, Gerald: "One Year's Advertisements." *British Medical Journal,* **1** 542 (1966).

The Cost of
Medicine Swallowing

Professor D. R. Laurence in his *Clinical Pharmacology* suggests that a doctor, before treating any patient with drugs, should make up his mind on the following five points:

1. *Whether he should interfere with the patient at all; and if so—*
2. *What alterations in the patient's condition he hopes to achieve.*
3. *That the drug he intends to use is capable of bringing this about.*
4. *What other effects the drug may have, and whether these effects may be harmful.*
5. *Whether the likelihood of benefit, and its importance, outweighs the likelihood of damage, and its importance.*

Using Professor Laurence's criteria, I have found that of 300 consecutive patients seen by me in a London general practice it was correct to prescribe a drug for only 45 of these patients. Actually, I found it quite impossible to reduce my prescription rate as low as that; to do so would have caused a waiting room rebellion. In England, the traditional need for medicines has become a social right.

Sir William Osler, the great Canadian physician, wrote:

Man has an inborn craving for medicines . . . it is really one of the most serious difficulties with which we have to contend.

In most countries of the Western world, either governments or insurance companies now pay a large chunk of the
cost of drugs. This has an effect on the kind of medicines
that doctors prescribe. The actual number of prescriptions
that they issue has not greatly increased, for doctors were
doling out prescriptions at an enormous rate long before the
inauguration of health insurance schemes. But the cost of
these prescriptions has certainly gone up. In the last 20
years, in countries which have health insurance schemes, the
cost of drugs has quadrupled.

Certainly, modern drugs are usually more expensive than
the simpler concoctions of 20 years ago. Yet a cheap drug can
sometimes be as effective as an expensive drug. But when
the state or the insurance company pays for the drugs, there
is no incentive for a doctor to prescribe a cheap drug, nor for
a patient to accept such a drug. Drug companies advertise
their proprietary products on which their profits are large.
Not surprisingly, their advertising is effective.

Therapeutic Largesse

Government health subsidies can be an expensive way of providing medicines. For instance, in Britain in 1967, when 100
aspirin could be bought over the counter for 12 cents, the cost
to the National Health Service of a doctor prescribing 25
tablets of the ten most commonly prescribed proprietary pain-
killers averaged 65 cents. In that year, the British National
Health Service spent (hospitals excluded) 16 million dollars
on these pain-killers. This expenditure was enough to have
supplied everyone in Britain, including babies, with 277 aspirin tablets, if these had been bought over the counter.

Proprietary analgesics often look appealing; they are usually nicely flavored, and they come in charming packages.
But the actual drugs they contain are no different from those
in cheaper pain killers marketed in simple glass bottles. It is
the gold and silver wrappings that are expensive, and the
patient who does not himself pay for the cost of drugs, is

usually only too willing to accept such glitter.

Under the National Health Service in Great Britain all drugs were once entirely free. But successive British governments have been trying to discourage the overconsumption of medicines and to reduce their enormous cost by introducing increasingly large prescription charges. Such prescription charges have not proved successful. Patients and doctors alike regard these charges as a tax on illness, and they retaliate by increasing the quantities on each prescription. The extra cost of these larger prescriptions eats up most of the money collected through prescription charges.

The British Government is considering making prescription charges proportional to the cost of the drugs supplied. Since some essential drugs are expensive, such a solution will certainly cause some sick people the kind of financial hardship that the National Health Service and other such schemes were designed to prevent. It might be more sensible if we stopped regarding all treatments as sacrosanct—if we stopped regarding all drugs as equally useful, and therefore equally deserving of public subsidy. Perhaps some drugs should be subsidized and others should not.

The United States is the country that spends the most on drugs. Its total drug bill for 1970 was 66 billion dollars. The majority of the drugs that were bought for this money did little or no good, and quite a lot of them did harm.

But not only do drugs often waste money, they also waste time. In the U.S. there is one family doctor for every 3,500 people. If the family doctor works a 44-hour week and takes a two-week vacation each year, he will work 2,200 hours yearly. Assuming that he has no other professional obligations, spends no time on the purely business administration of his practice, never goes to refresher courses, and never gets stuck in traffic jams, the doctor will have 38 minutes *a year* to spend on each patient. A patient who takes even three minutes each month to collect prescriptions for his favorite sleeping tablets or reducing pills uses up nearly all his fair share of doctor time. Too little time is left over for more useful care.

Indeed, doctors are so busy prescribing that they have little time for anything else. In Britain, for instance, each family doctor in 1970 wrote an average of 12,900 prescriptions. This means that during their office hours British doctors must write prescriptions at the rate of one prescription every six minutes.

In spite of the rush in which they work, family doctors can often tell at a glance who is sick and who is not; they can quickly spot one who is seriously sick and send him to a hospital. But serious disease can be overlooked because doctors are so busy handing out prescriptions that they do not have time to decide what disease, if any, they are actually treating. Fortunately, human beings are usually self-repairing. Usually it makes not the slightest difference what treatment the patient is given. He gets better anyway.

Drug Hoarding

Even in the midst of today's enthusiasm for medication, many patients fail to take their medicines. One recent British study showed that a third of the patients failed to take prescribed antibiotics or took them in a desultory way. Among the chronically ill, the percentage of defaulters is even higher. Only between a third and a half of tubercular and psychiatric outpatients actually take the medicines that they are prescribed.

Even addictive drugs are not always taken regularly, and patients store them up as squirrels store up nuts. In one 10-day period, a coroner's officer investigating sudden deaths in North London filled a gallon jar with pills, mostly hypnotics, collected from ordinary homes.

Too often a few pills are taken from a new bottle, which is then relegated to the back of the bathroom medicine cabinet, where it awaits the next adventurous child that comes along. In some English cities, more children die each year from medication poisoning than from measles, polio, rheumatic fever, scarlet fever, and tuberculosis combined. Aspirin-containing tablets, barbiturates, and iron tablets are the poisons that kill the most children.

Some patients play Russian roulette with the drugs pre-scribed for them. Ohio State University Hospital followed up on 40 of its outpatients to find out how well they were obey-ing the doctors' instructions. It was found that 90 percent were making some mistake with their medication, and that 20 percent were either doubling or trebling prescribed quan-

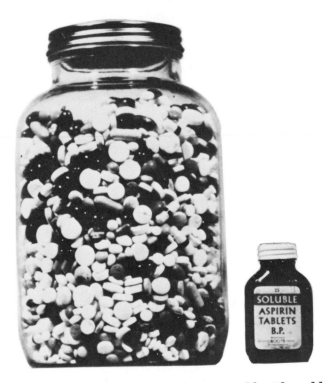

"Psychiatric drugs" can cause a lot of trouble. The tablets in this gallon jar are mostly hypnotics. They were all collected within 10 days by a coroner's officer investigating sudden deaths in North London.

tities *by continuing to take medication prescribed previously,* perhaps by another doctor.

Many drugs are potent, and doubling or trebling the dosage may be dangerous. Digitalis, useful in the treatment of congestive heart failure, is often given to the elderly. But digitalis is very poisonous, and about 60 percent of the toxic dose is required to achieve any therapeutic effect. Therefore, if an elderly person absentmindedly doubles the number of tablets he should be taking, he is more likely to benefit his heirs than himself.

As people age, they develop more diseases; and therefore, they collect more bottles of pills. I counted 36 unidentified bottles of pills by the bedside of one confused and dying old lady. None of her family knew which pills were for what, but every few hours they gave her some more. In the process, they used the good domestic principle that nearly empty bottles should be used up first.

Lax Controls

So infinite appears to be our faith in the unalloyed beneficence of our favorite pills, that not only do we forget that people often use these pills in most extraordinary ways, but we also seem willing to overlook how many of these pills never actually reach those for whom they were intended.

Drugs of addiction cost money. Because the respectable use them, the unrespectable can filch them. On both sides of the Atlantic, thefts from drugstores and their suppliers become more frequent. The U.S. Food and Drug Administration has estimated that more than 25 tons of legally manufactured amphetamine find their way into illegal channels. This is sufficient to supply each person in the United States with 14 amphetamine tablets a year.

British hospitals are notoriously careless with their addictive drugs. Patients are frequently prescribed sleeping pills; hospitals, therefore, stock very large quantities of sleeping tablets. A survey I made in one large London mental hospital showed that only one-third of the night sedatives that left the dispensary were legitimately administered to patients; the other two-thirds remained unaccounted for.

If doctors prescribed only useful drugs for their patients, and having done so, then encouraged their patients actually to take them, health insurance might be less expensive and many of us would be healthier.

SOURCES

British Medical Association Advisory Panel: *Health Services Financing*. London: British Medical Association, 1970.

Department of Health and Social Security: *Annual Report for the Year 1968*. London: Her Majesty's Stationery Office, 1969.

————: *Annual Report for the Year 1970*. London: Her Majesty's Stationery Office, 1971.

Dubnow, M. H., and Burchell, H. B.: "A Comparison of Digitalis Intoxication in Two Separate Periods." *Annals of Internal Medicine*, **62** 956 (1965).

Eimerl, T. S., and Pearson, R. J. C.: "Working Time in General Practice: How General Practitioners Use Their Time." *British Medical Journal*, **2** 1549 (1966).

Griffith, John: "A Study of Illicit Amphetamine Drug Traffic in Oklahoma City." *American Journal of Psychiatry*, **123** 560 (1966).

Hemphill, R. E.: "Unreliability of Psychiatric Patients in Following Prescribing Instructions." *Journal of College of General Practitioners*, **65** (1966).

Laurence, D. R.: *Clinical Pharmacology*. London: J. & A. Churchill, 1966.

Lown, B., and Levine, S. A.: "Current Concepts in Digitalis Therapy." *New England Journal of Medicine*, **250** 771 and 819 (1954).

Luntz, G. R. W., and Austin, R.: "New Stick Test for P.A.S. in Urine." *British Medical Journal*, **1** 1679 (1960).

Malahy, Bernadine: "The Effect of Instruction and Labeling on the Number of Medication Errors Made by Patients at Home." *American Journal of Hospital Pharmacology*, **23** 283 (1966).

Matthew, H.: "Poisoning in the Home by Medicaments." *British Medical Journal*, **2** 788 (1966).

Ministry of Health: *Annual Report for the Year 1950*. London: Her Majesty's Stationery Office, 1951.

————: Committee on Cost of Prescribing: *Final Report*. London: Her Majesty's Stationery Office, 1959.

Nicolson, W. A.: "Collection of Unwanted Drugs from Private Homes." *British Medical Journal,* **3** 730 (1967).

Porter, A. M.: "Drug Defaulting in a General Practice." *British Medical Journal,* **1** 218 (1969).

U.S. Bureau of the Census: *Statistical Abstract of the U.S.A.* Washington, D.C.: Government Printing Office, 1971.

Webb, S. and W.: *The State and the Doctor.* London: Longman's & Co., 1910.

Wilcox, D. R. C., Gillan, R., and Hare, E. H.: "Do Psychiatric Out-Patients Take Their Drugs?" *British Medical Journal,* **2** 790 (1965).

World Health Organization: "The Consumption of Drugs." *WHO Chronicle,* **24** 68 (1970).

Rival Insights to the Mind

Rational behavior does not come in bottles. Psychotherapy is a treatment which aims to teach people to live their lives more effectively. Learning to do this is no different from learning fluent French or gourmet cookery. It requires an industrious pupil, and it is made easier by the help of a skilled teacher. But learning is hard work.

The term "self-improver" has been used to describe anyone who at any time after leaving school, has taken any course of instruction, be it only knitting. Self-improvers are in the minority; for instance, only 30 percent of the people of Britain are self-improvers. Certainly among middle-class Americans self-improvement is close to being a national habit, yet probably fewer than one-third of *all* adults on either side of the Atlantic bother to learn even simple new skills. Probably even fewer are interested in the difficult task of learning new skills for living their lives more effectively.

Sometimes, of course, the necessity to learn these new skills is forced upon people. The "rock bottom" described by Alcoholics Anonymous may be such an occasion. An alcoholic who finally loses family, friends, possessions, and self-respect hits rock bottom. If he decides the game is not worth the candle, he joins AA, learns to cope with life without alcohol, and stays sober.

Talk treatments work if the patient is prepared to work hard at getting better; and if the teacher—be he doctor, convert, counselor, saint, or psychologist—is skilled at his job. But many people do not want to get better, and what many teachers teach leads to disease, not to health.

The Efficacy of Psychotherapy

It is no simple matter to measure the effectiveness of psychotherapy. H. J. Eysenck, professor of psychology at the Maudsley Hospital, London, concludes that:

> When untreated neurotic control groups are compared with experimental groups of neurotic patients treated by means of psychotherapy, both groups recover to approximately the same extent.
>
> When soldiers who have suffered a neurotic breakdown and have not received psychotherapy are compared with soldiers who have received psychotherapy, the chances of the two groups returning to duty are approximately equal.
>
> Civilian neurotics who are treated by psychotherapy recover or improve to approximately the same extent as similar neurotics receiving no psychotherapy.
>
> Children suffering from emotional disorders and treated by psychotherapy recover or improve to approximately the same extent as similar children not receiving psychotherapy.

Eysenck is certainly the analysts' bad dream. He found that *the more analytically oriented the therapy, the lower the recovery rate.* In fact, psychoanalysis actually delays recovery. Spontaneous remission of symptoms occurs in 72 percent of cases. Improvement after psychoanalytical treatment occurs in only 44 percent of cases.

Two-thirds of neurotic patients recover or improve to a marked extent within two years of the onset of their illness, whether they are treated by psychotherapy or not. Professor Eysenck comments that from the point of view of the neurotic these figures are encouraging; "from the point of view of the psychotherapist they can hardly be called favorable to his claims."

Yet the efficacy of psychotherapy is seldom questioned. It is simply accepted by conventional wisdom as a major bulwark in the fight against mental illness and social collapse. One of the most thorough of the few controlled studies that have been made into the effectiveness of psychotherapy was conducted in the Cambridge-Somerville area of Massachusetts.

Between 1937 and 1945, a large-scale treatment effort was directed toward the prevention of delinquency, by guidance, counseling, and psychotherapy of underprivileged boys between the ages of six and 10. Six-hundred-fifty boys were chosen for the experiment because their social backgrounds indicated they were likely to become deliquents. The boys were then individually matched by age, intelligence, school grade, delinquency rating, and ethnic and socioeconomic background. One of each pair was assigned by the toss of a coin either to the treatment group or to the control group. In this way, two groups of boys were obtained whose chances of becoming delinquent were equal.

The 325 boys in the treatment group were assigned to counselors and received individual counseling or psychotherapy for periods of two to eight years. All counseling and psychotherapy was withheld from the control group. After the treatment was finished, the counselors listed two-thirds of the treated boys as having "substantially benefited" from the program. More than half of these boys stated that they had been helped.

Offenses committed by the boys of the two groups and their appearances in court were then compared. The boys in the treatment group had committed 264 offenses; those in the control group 218. The treatment group boys appeared in court 96 times; the control group boys only 92 times.

Although most of the counselors and their clients regarded the psychotherapy program as having been useful, the goals of the psychotherapy were not achieved. The treated boys remained as delinquent in their behavior as the untreated boys. With psychotherapy, as with pills, the more closely the effects of treatment are compared to the effects of no treatment, the less effective treatment is found to be.

Freud, the Forgiving Father

It is beyond argument that Freud's theories have had an enormous influence upon psychiatric thinking; but the usefulness of Freudian psychotherapy is open to argument.

Dr. Alex Comfort has dubbed doctors "the anxiety makers." I seek to make you tremble each time you lay a hand upon a pill—a hundred years ago it would have been a hand upon your genitals. The work of Sigmund Freud has at least made the latter more comfortable for you.

Dr. Henry Maudsley endowed the hospital that bears his name; it is now the leading psychiatric institute in England. Dr. Maudsley was certainly one of the more intelligent and enlightened psychiatrists of the 19th century. He probably would even have agreed with the contentions of this book; for in 1879, he was writing about the "propriety" of the free use of sedatives in the treatment of insanity. He suggested that it be considered "seriously whether the putting of nerve cells in the patients' brains into chemical restraint did really benefit them." He would not have liked the barbiturates, nor Valium, nor Librium, nor any of the other drugs with which today's psychiatrists douse the brains of their patients.

But Dr. Maudsley, like his contemporaries, rode the popular Victorian hobbyhorse—he believed in the evils of masturbation. In 1865, he gave a lecture to the Harveian Society on this then fashionable subject. Some extracts from his lecture will illustrate the kind of hobbyhorse from which Freud unseated his medical colleagues, and will demonstrate nicely what Dr. Comfort means by anxiety-making:

> *The first class of patients of this kind to which I may direct attention is that comprising youths of about 18 years of age. They are brought for medical advice by their parents or other relatives, because they are not*

doing any good at the business to which they have been put, and their masters complain that they can make nothing of them. They show no interest, and put no energy, in what they are set to do; they are forgetful, moody, careless, abstracted, perhaps muttering to themselves, and waste a long time in doing badly very simple things, or fail to do them . . . meanwhile at home they are selfish, irritable, exacting, very deceitful, and passionate; they are entirely wanting in reverence for their parents, or in proper feeling for others; and their pretensions are outrageous. They themselves by no means admit that they give any just ground of complaint; but make some excuse for their conduct by putting the blame of it on persons or circumstances, or deny it altogether.

It is always so: always some excuse for failure and faults, which are entirely in themselves—for a course of conduct really due to a sort of moral insanity.

If you question these youths about their vicious habits, or charge them with it, you are not likely to get an acknowledgement of it; the most they will admit probably is that they have erred once or twice; but they will deny solemnly that they are continuing the habit. There is no faith to be put in their most solemn assertations, their moral nature being thoroughly vitiated. A later and still worse stage at which these degenerate beings arrive is one of moody and morose self-absorption, and of extreme loss of mental power. The body is usually much emaciated, notwithstanding they eat well; and though they often last for a longer period than might be thought possible, they finally totter on to death through a complete prostration of the entire system, if they are not carried off by some intercurrent disease.

Such then is the natural history of the physical and mental degeneracy produced in men by self-

*abuse. It is a miserable picture of human degrada-
tion, but it is not overcharged. When we meet in
practice with its painful features, we know what had
been the cause of the disease, and what must be its
inevitable termination. I have nothing to add con-
cerning treatment; once the habit is formed, and the
mind has positively suffered from it, the victim is less
able to control what is more difficult of control, and
there would be almost as much hope of the Ethiopian
changing his skin, or the leopard its spots, as of his
abandoning the vice. I have no faith in the employment of physical means to check what has become a
serious mental disease; the sooner he sinks to his de-
graded rest the better for himself, and the better for
the world which is well rid of him.*

I do not suppose young men have changed their sexual
habits much in the last 100 years. If you endow a mental hospital, this is at least one way of ensuring that there will be a lot
of anxious people to fill it.

Freud, by his remarkable perspicacity and strong courage,
turned the searchlight of scientific inquiry onto human sexuality. The spell of reticence was broken; the fear that blinkered
our Victorian forefathers receded. Human beings almost
started to enjoy their sex lives, and doctors almost stopped

*The "meagre" appearance, inflammation of the eyes, and total
relaxation of both testicles, all due to "self-pollution." The
pictures are from* The Silent Friend, *a medical manual for the
public published in 1853 by R. and L. Perry & Co. This book
devoted 75 pages to the disastrous effects of self-pollution on
the mind and body. R. and L. Perry & Co. happened to be the
manufacturers of Perry's pills, a purifying specific which
protected against the effects of masturbation. They sold these
pills at an enormous price in England, the European continent, and the U.S.A.*

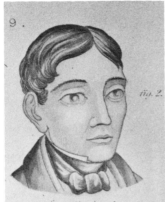

9.

fig. 2.

Spermatorrhœal
Opthalmia consequent through Onanism

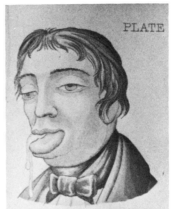

PLATE

The meagre appearance of the features
through Onanism.

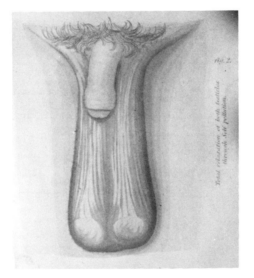

fig. 2.

Total relaxation of both testicles
through Self pollution.

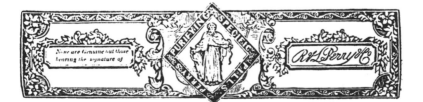

None are Genuine but those
bearing the signature of

R L Perry &Co

being prigs. Professional criticism was reserved for those parents who by their repressive behavior enhanced the superegos of their children. For good or bad, permissive society was born.

Freud's genius also devised a system of mind that, for the last half century, has served as an explanation of human behavior. Were he alive today, Freud would almost certainly be the first to agree that his explanation of the workings of the mind has proved to be very lopsided. Unfortunately, the glitter of his theories discouraged others from looking for a more realistic understanding of how the mind works, and why we behave in the ways we do.

Freudians envisage a volcano of repressed sexual desire, shabby guilt, and frustrated love rumbling in the depths of the mind. This volcano of psychopathology may erupt into an explosion of mental illness or may gently belch forth with symptoms of neurotic disorder. Determined removal of such symptoms merely causes a further breach in the frail crust of sanity. One symptom will be exchanged for another; and the new one may be worse. Only by the understanding of its contents can the volcano be tamed and its energies usefully released. Without such understanding, the individual is powerless in the face of this destructive energy.

Understanding and cure, the Freudians teach, can be gained only through analysis. This means that if you are mentally unwell and cannot afford analysis, you might as well not bother to try to get better. You will stay sick anyway, for the cause of the disorder is beyond your reach.

The New Biology

Freud had the disadvantage of working in a factual vacuum. Much more is now known about the biology of behavior and learning. Ethology, the science of animal behavior, has greatly broadened the scientific backdrop against which human behavior can be studied. Writers such as Desmond Morris, Konrad Lorenz, and Robert Ardrey have popularized an understanding of human behavior in terms of our more furry contemporaries.

Patterns of animal behavior, like the shapes of their bodies, develop during the evolution of their species. Inherited behavior is called instinct. Instinct may direct tightly predetermined patterns of behavior. In the higher species of the animal kingdom, instinct may direct a predisposition to behave in a certain way. It is hotly argued whether human behavior can sometimes be ascribed to instinct.

Robert Ardrey has argued a substantial case for at least some part of human aggression being derived from an instinct to protect group territory. We do not hate Catholics, Protestants, Jews, blacks, whites, browns, the Irish, the Americans, or any other popular hate group because we have been frustrated as infants and are filled to the brim with unconscious aggression, but because group identity and alien-group hostility were once useful survival mechanisms of our species.

If Ardrey is right, then it is more likely that people will learn to live without war by the clear recognition that they fight for fun, the fun of gratifying their instincts. Hoping that political leaders will diminish their aggressive impulses by rummaging around among their infantile memories may be the solution of psychoanalysts, but if Ardrey is right that kind of therapy will hardly avail. Since psychoanalysts have remained as belligerent as the rest of us, their solution to the problem of war and aggression never gained much credibility.

However, nor are the views of the "new biologists" accepted by everybody. Ashley Montagu, for one, has led a heated attack upon these new theories in *Man and Aggression*. It may be difficult to disentangle the rights and wrongs of all the arguments; but when an academic starts getting very angry, one can at least be pretty certain that another academic has invaded his territory.

Sexual Behavior

In spite of the research done on animal and human behavior, we still really know very little about the causes of normal or abnormal behavior. Experiments with rats show that sex hormones given before or soon after birth can permanently modify the sexual behavior of these creatures. One injection of a male hormone given immediately after birth to a female rat will make her subsequent sexual behavior resemble that of a male. It is now believed that there is a critical period during the development of the mammalian brain during which it is susceptible to permanent alteration through sex hormones.

It is not known why men and women develop male and female patterns of sexual behavior. Possibly such behavior patterns are entirely the product of human culture and individual experience. Possibly they are, at least in part, determined by instinct, or by imprinting mechanisms operating at crucial periods in the individual's development, or by the actions of hormones on the developing brain before birth.

Certain drugs interfere with the action of male hormone upon the developing brain. Dr. John Money of Johns Hopkins has gathered evidence from studies with the rats and monkeys that indicates that certain sleeping pills, an antibiotic called actinomycin B, and some psychoactive drugs can cause transsexuality. He suggests that the normal programming of a male foetus brain may be distorted if the pregnant mother takes these drugs, which may predispose her son to have a problem with gender identity. It may be that a mother whose doctor gives her barbiturates when she is pregnant will have not only a stupid son, but one who likes wearing drag as well.

The hormone progesterone is sometimes prescribed by doctors to pregnant women in an attempt to prevent miscarriage. A study of a group of girls whose mothers had been treated with this masculinizing hormone showed that they were more "butch" than normal. Rather surprisingly, progesterone, in contrast to the barbiturates, was also found to increase intelligence; and the girls of the study had higher than expected IQ's. Even for scientists, sex still retains its mysteries.

What is it that makes a man feel comfortable and only truly himself when he wears a sanitary napkin and can imagine himself with a period? Why is it that although everybody agrees that it is a man's world, there are long queues of men requesting sex change operations? The possible explanations are many; but doctors do not really know the cause of this kind of deviation, just as they do not know the causes of most of our other abnormal behavior. Still less do they know what to do to put such behavior right.

This does not mean, of course, that there are no treatments for the mind. There are many; and although these treatments are often based on contradictory suppositions about the workings of the mind and the body, all these treatments are claimed by the doctors who use them to work.

Which Treatment Will Work?

Psychoanalysis remains, especially in the United States, the most prestigious treatment, and certainly the most expensive. In its salad days, psychoanalysis was used for the treatment of the common sexual deviations: fetishism, homosexuality, wrong gender identity, sadomasochism. Most patients with such problems completed their analysis retaining the same oddities with which they started. Exploring repressed interests and desires sometimes bestowed upon some patients even more aberrations. Today, Freudian psychoanalysis is no longer generally accepted as the panacea for these problems.

The anxious and the depressed now form the bulk of the analyst's clientele. It is the people with these discomforts who are most ready to commit themselves to the expense and the time that analysis involves. To be allowed to explore intimate feelings and ideas with a sympathetic and intelligent person is, of course, likely to lead to interesting conversation. Many people find this in itself both rewarding and useful.

But the usefulness of disentangling the hypothetical causes of symptoms is more questionable, since this often seems to delay recovery. Psychoanalysis can have exactly the same disadvantage as treatment by pills: the patient postpones making an effort to cope with the problems of his life until the treatment begins to work. It often does not.

For hospital psychiatry, analytical theory has proved disastrous. Analytical theory teaches that disturbed behavior is the product of unconscious conflict, that removal of symptoms merely results in their substitution by others, and that treatment is only to be achieved by the resolution of the unconscious conflict.

But often such conflict cannot be resolved. When a mental hospital patient steals from other patients, or by anti-social behavior demands staff attention, it is customary to regard him as deprived of parental love. When he smashes windows, it is because of unresolved aggression. The resolution of such hypothetical unconscious conflicts is beyond the capacity both of most patients and most hospitals. Yet the theory subsists.

Many psychiatrists regard it as useless or even harmful to deal directly with such anti-social behavior; so willy-nilly, hospitals put up with such behavior with as good grace as they can muster. Often patients, like children for whom no limits to unacceptable behavior have been set, test their guardians to the limit of endurance. It is not surprising that such misbehaving patients are medicated until they are too sleepy to be bad. The problem is shelved.

This situation reaches the ultimate in absurdity when the drugs used for this purpose are addictive. Bad behavior, then, becomes the best way of insuring an adequate supply of the wanted drugs.

Freudian "determinism" when used as a basis for social conduct only determines chaos. It is no longer the individual who determines his behavior but the innumerable forces of his past: "Doctor, if I only know what caused my problem, I would be able to do something about it." This, under the guidance of modern psychiatry, is now accepted patient philosophy. Since the cause of the problem usually remains obscure to both the patient and the doctor, the patient can continue to cling to his problem, and persist in his behavior.

Living without one's problem is hard work. It becomes necessary to find something else to put in the place of the problem; this requires a creative effort. Many people, therefore, prefer to stick with their familiar problems; the determinism of psychoanalysis provides a good excuse for doing just that. Teaching people that they are not responsible for their behavior is not useful.

The Behaviorist Approach

After Eysenck had demonstrated to all those who would believe him that Freudian psychotherapy was useless, he and his co-workers in London developed behaviorist theory and applied it to the treatment of neurosis and anti-social behavior. Joseph Wolpe in the United States worked along parallel lines. Behaviorists such as Eysenck and Wolpe regard neurotic, and sometimes even psychotic, behavior as learned bad habits.

What is learned can be unlearned. The behaviorists would make use of the modern learning theories they have developed in their laboratory experiments. Behavior therapy is an up-and-coming treatment, especially fashionable among youth and enthusiastic Ph.D. psychologists. Psychologists do not like being left with their laboratory rats while psychiatrists make off with profitable patients. Patients, after all, often pay for their treatment; rats do not. Behavior therapy enables psychologists to compete with psychiatrists upon more than equal terms in the treatment of mental illness. For psychologists with their rats have been trained in these particular methods, and psychiatrists have not.

Grandma probably would not understand the language of learning theory, but she would have no difficulty with its principles. She practiced them for years.

Pavlov, his dog, his bell, and his conditioned reflex form the why and the wherefore of the behaviorists' activities. Pavlov rang a bell and gave a dog a bone. After he had done this about 40 times, the dog salivated whenever he heard the bell. He had been conditioned.

Dr. J. B. Watson, the distinguished behavioral psychologist, conducted what has become one of the best known ex-

periments. Eleven-month-old little Albert was fond of animals. Dr. Watson showed him a white rat. Whenever little
Albert reached out for the rat, Dr. Watson made a loud noise
behind little Albert by banging on an iron bar. Little Albert
developed a phobia toward white rats, and indeed, toward all
furry animals; he had been conditioned to be frightened by
them. Dr. Watson was unkind to little Albert; but behaviorists in general try to be more helpful.

Reinforcement, the psychologists teach, is anything that
increases the probability that a response will recur. Little
Jimmy finds his grandma's eyeglasses for her after she has forgotten for the nth time where she left them. She rewards him
with a bar of chocolate. The chocolate increases the probability that he will give the glasses to her the next time he
finds them. Grandma is practicing positive reinforcement.

But Jimmy now steals Grandma's apples. She, with her
glasses safely on, catches him, and she beats him with her
umbrella. Psychologists, when they practice "aversive reinforcement," prefer painful electric shocks. Grandma and the
psychologists sometimes meet with success. However, experiments in both animal and human learning show that positive
reinforcement is considerably more effective than is aversive
reinforcement. The chocolate accomplishes more than the
umbrella.

One day, while Jimmy was again stealing apples, aversive
reinforcement not having been that effective, he was again
caught, this time by his nasty sister's nasty horse. The horse
bit him. Jimmy, as did little Albert with the white rat, developed a phobia of horses. He would not go near a field in which
there was one, and he also was afraid of other animals. Psychologists would say that his fear had "generalized," and that
now he had developed a whole "hierarchy" of fears. His nasty
sister's nasty horse topped the list. Then came other horses,
then cows, then pigs; he did not even like dogs very much any
more.

His helpful grandma now gave Jimmy a puppy. He soon
became fond of it. She held his hand, and she took him to

see pigs. Another day, she bought him an ice cream cone and she took him to see some cows. Psychologists say that "if a response inhibitory of anxiety can be made to occur in the presence of the anxiety-evoking stimuli, it will weaken the bond between these stimuli and the anxiety." Grandma with her ice cream cone was practicing reciprocal inhibition and "counterconditioning." Jimmy soon wanted to see the cows being milked.

After this, it was not difficult to persuade him to visit the horses. Jimmy even learned to pat his nasty sister's nasty horse. Grandma had worked through Jimmy's hierarchy of fears. Psychologists call this "systematic desensitization."

When Jimmy grew up, he took to wearing his grandma's bra and girdle. This stretched both her clothes and her patience. He was sent to a doctor who practiced behavior therapy.

The doctor told him to dress in his favorite garments, and then gave him a drug to make him feel sick. This was repeated many times. Jimmy learned through this to respond to the bra and the girdle, not with thrill and delight, but with fear and discomfort. He has been conditioned to dislike them. Jimmy has been turned off. If she had faith in the behaviorist's treatment, Grandma could relax again.

Positive Reinforcement

The concepts of behaviorists are now being widely applied; and, perhaps, they are sometimes useful. Some mental hospitals have found a simple and rather effective way of reducing socially unacceptable behavior: they reward virtue.

In most mental hospitals, patients gain status by their eccentricities and learn to gain attention by madness or badness. Under a behaviorist-oriented regime, the staff is trained not to reward with attention patients who behave madly or badly. If a patient approaches a member of the staff in a normal and pleasant way, the staff member responds. If he approaches with mad talk, the staff member turns away and ignores him. The patient is thus rewarded for his acceptable behavior, and punished for his unacceptable behavior. And patient behavior improves.

Positive reinforcement is the theoretical basis for what is called a "token economy." Teodora Ayllon and Nathan Azrin noticed that educators, mothers, and industry all provide incentives in order to modify behavior. They decided to try doing the same in a mental hospital. Working in the Anna State Hospital in Illinois, they pioneered their system in the early 1960s. It is now being used with success in other mental hospitals.

Small behavioral improvement goals are set for patients. As each goal is achieved, the patient is rewarded with a token. The tokens can be used to buy food, cigarettes, and privileges within the hospital. Thus, patients are provided with something to work for. Even the behavior of extremely deteriorated and incontinent patients sometimes improves; and many long-stay patients have become competent enough to be discharged.

B. F. Skinner is also enthusiastic about such modification techniques, and his views are well respected among many university psychologists. Dr. Skinner is a radical behaviorist, and not only does he have no truck with the unconscious conflicts of the Freudians, but he has even done away with human free will. He regards our behaviors as a consequence of the "contingencies of reinforcement" to which we are exposed.

Translated into ordinary English, this means that he regards our behavior as only a series of responses to the world around us. We cannot freely decide to behave in a better way; we can only do so if there is some payoff for such behavior. We are helpless puppets of our environment, and our behavior can be improved for the better only by arranging for the environment to reinforce us in more appropriate ways. His critics, especially those familiar with professional helpers, are left wondering who is going to do the rearranging.

Psychiatrists, psychologists, and sociologists disagree on just about everything that can be disagreed upon. They have,

however, one thing in common. They like to devise and prop-
agate new theories for the understanding, explanation, control, and improvement of our behavior. We have defeated
them. Behavior is much too complicated to be comfortably
encompassed by any of their theories. Nevertheless, their theories do provide simple insights into what we do and why we
do it.

As a practical way of dealing with people and their often
wayward behavior, Freud's theories turned out to be disastrous, and the schemes of the behaviorists more useful. Behaviorists at least sustain the hope that we can always learn
to do better.

Return to Freedom

Both analysts and behaviorists are deterministic: they believe
that people are forced to behave in the way they do because of
their past. But some psychiatrists are now giving patients back
their freedom. These psychiatrists are devising new, and perhaps more robust, schemes for the understanding of behavior.
Their humanistic approach claims that people behave in the
way they do because this is the way they choose to behave. No
one is a helpless creature of circumstance.

Mr. Jones is tired of feeling that he is a friendless failure. He would much prefer to be popular. Mr. Jones therefore decides to break with reality. He calls himself Napoleon.

Mr. Smith is not a good businessman, though he believes
he is. He maintains his companies lose money because the
Jews are plotting against him. This belief both excuses his
failure, and gives him the added status of being important
enough to be plotted against.

Grandmother insists on living in her childhood. Perhaps
it is not only arterial sclerosis that makes her do so. She finds
her useless life in the living graveyard of a nursing home de-
testable, and she prefers to return to the years when she was
young and pretty and the apple of her mother's eye.

If life becomes too unrewarding, if the prospects of the

future are too intolerably dismal, if a man has never learned to cope with the inevitable difficulties of living, if a man is incapacitated by brain disease or ill health, then a break with reality may become an acceptable choice. And sometimes failure is easier to choose than success.

If the achievement of success is too difficult, if a man cannot find for himself a meaningful niche in life, if he finds life horribly difficult, then failure becomes acceptable.

The Responsibility for Sickness

A man may choose to remain hopeless, helpless, and in need. By failure, he avoids the hard work of success; he disowns responsibility for the world around him, and he gets looked after. Dr. William Glasser, the author of *Reality Therapy*, suggests that mental illness should not be regarded as an illness but as irresponsible behavior, irresponsible because it entails the conscious decision to break with the requirements and standards of everyday life.

If we regard all illness as something that just happens to a person and believe he can do nothing himself to make himself well, then kindness dictates that we must do what we can to support the sick person in his sick and sorry state. Certainly this may sometimes be true. Nevertheless, by regarding all sickness as beyond an individual's responsibility, we often help to establish the sick person in his chosen position of helplessness. He stays sick.

By placing responsibility for sickness upon the ill, we at least make him free to do something about it. He can then, if he so chooses, accept help in finding a more constructive way of living.

SOURCES

Arai, Y., and Gorski, R. A.: "Protection Against the Neural Organizing Effect of Exogenous Androgen in the Neonatal Female Rat." *Endocrinology*, **82** 1005 (1968).

Ardrey, Robert: *African Genesis*. New York: Atheneum Publishers, 1961.

———: *The Social Contract*. New York: Atheneum Publishers, 1970.

———: *The Territorial Imperative*. New York: Atheneum Publishers, 1966.

Ayllon, Teodora, and Azrin, Nathan: *The Token Economy: A Motivational System for Therapy and Rehabilitation*. New York: Appleton-Century-Crofts, 1968.

Comfort, Alex: *The Anxiety Makers*. London: Thomas Nelson & Son, 1967.

Eysenck, H. J.: *The Effects of Psychotherapy*. New York: International Science Press, 1966.

———: "The Effects of Psychotherapy: An Evaluation." *Journal of Consulting and Clinical Psychology*, **16** 319 (1952).

Gadpaille, Warren J.: "Research Into the Physiology of Maleness and Femaleness." *Archives of General Psychiatrics*, **26** 193 (1972).

Glasser, William: *Reality Therapy*. New York: Harper and Row, 1965.

Goldfoot, D. A., Feder, H. H., and Goy, R. W.: "Development of Bisexuality in the Male Rat Treated Neonatally with Androstenedione." *Journal of Comparative Physiology and Psychology*. **67** 41 (1969).

Lorenz, Konrad: *On Aggression*. London: Methuen, 1966.

———: *King Solomon's Ring*. London: Methuen, 1952.

Luttge, G. W., and Whalen, R. E.: "Partial Defeminization." *Life Science*, **8** 1003 (1969).

Maudsley, Henry: "Illustrations of a Variety of Insanity." *Journal of Mental Science*, **14** 149 (1968).

———: *The Pathology of the Mind.* London: Macmillan & Co., 1895.

Montagu, Ashley M. F.: *Man and Aggression.* London: Oxford University Press, 1968.

Morris, Desmond: *The Human Zoo.* London: Jonathan Cape, 1969.

———: *The Naked Ape.* London: Jonathan Cape, 1967.

Skinner, B. F.: *Beyond Freedom and Dignity.* New York: Alfred A. Knopf, Inc., 1971.

Tenber, Hans-Lukas, and Powers, Edwin: "Evaluating Therapy in a Delinquency Program." *Research Publications of the Association for the Research in Nervous and Mental Diseases,* **31** 138 (1953); Baltimore: Williams and Wilkins Co., 1953.

Watson, J. B., and Rayner, R.: "Conditioned Emotional Reaction." *Journal of Experimental Psychology,* **3** 14 (1920).

Wolpe, Joseph, and Lazarus, Arnold A.: *Behavior Therapy Techniques.* New York: Pergamon Press, 1968.

The Uses of Sickness

A bus runs you over. Your hip is broken. You go into a hospital. You were an independent, though sometimes absentminded, adult. Now you are helpless. Your leg is strung to a beam above your head. It hurts to move, and you cannot sit up. You have to be fed and bedpanned. Your days were full, and now they are empty. The thought of two months in bed is devastating. All is black.

Yet the days slip by. The ward routine grows pleasing. Meals appear with calm regularity. The nurses are pretty, and it is nice to be catered to. You feel at home. You like the easy life. You could live like this forever. Soon you are shouting at the nurse if she is slow with the bedpan, and you have a temper tantrum if the soup is cold. You have regressed.

But the two months pass. The surgeon removes your leg splint and buxom physiotherapists pull you out of bed. Soon you are walking on crutches. A month later, you can walk without them. You are back at work. You are once again an independent adult.

Behavior Regression

Serious and incapacitating illness is almost invariably associated with regression of behavior to that of an earlier level of psychological development. On recovery from illness, most of us manage to mature again quite quickly.

For some, recovery is not so simple. There are advantages in being sick. If these advantages are large, recovery is more difficult. Somehow the leg stays weak, the crutches are difficult to manage, the limp produces backache. It is uncomfortable to walk. It is necessary to stay at home.

We easily get stuck at a dependent level of behavior. The first 15 years or so of our lives, loving parents make us secure and comfortable. During our most impressionable years, we learn how soothing it is to be looked after. It will always come easy to us. Perhaps all of us, but especially those who have been looked after too much or too little, will continue to hanker for care from others for the rest of our lives.

The rebellious years of adolescence leave most of us standing rather precariously upon our own two feet. Independence is a struggle. Finding a way to earn a living, finding somewhere to live, finding someone to live with, and finding a reason to live can be hard work. Justified by illness, many of us are prepared to swap the hard work of independence for the easy comfort of dependency.

Sickness has its uses. It can, for instance, provide status and love. Even the Prince Regent, the son of the English King who lost his American colonies, who because of his elegance is still known as "the first gentleman of Europe," often had himself bled so as to look pale and interesting. He cut his wrists to make Mrs. Fitzherbert love him.

Once women had theological doubts to win the attentions of their priests; now they have interesting psychological traumata to win the attentions of their doctors. Sickness wins attention, and often the sick member of the family hogs it all.

Sickness excuses failure and provides the right to be looked after. The monotony of work can be avoided and tiresome responsibilities shelved. A doctor's statement can be a passport in the modern welfare state to sick pay, better housing, home assistance, meals on wheels, and many other useful services.

Compensation Neurosis

People stay sick for a lot of reasons. But the man whose leg was broken by a bus and who believes it was the bus driver's fault is in serious trouble. He has a grievance, and he broods upon injustice. The bus company caused the accident: they must be made to pay. He has developed compensation neurosis.

Because the process of the law is slow, an injured person must nurture his sense of injury for a very long time. When at long last damages are paid, he is often so entrenched in a life of psychological invalidism that it is no longer easy for him to recover. Ill health and health are often just habits of mind.

If DOMP describes the diseases of medical practice caused by doctors and their good intentions, then perhaps DOLP should be used to describe the *Diseases of Legal Practice* caused by lawyers and legislators in their quest for "justice."

Industrial accidents provide the most fruitful source of compensation neurosis. Let us take California as a prime example. There, as in most modern communities, the law seeks to provide an injured employee with the best medical aid possible, to compensate him for loss of earnings, and to avoid involvement in litigation. Nevertheless, lawyers have turned compensation claims into big business, and the defense seldom wins.

Jeremiah Crawley, a Californian legal expert on compensation, writes in his *Lamentations of a Jeremiah* that

> *the injured employee is not always thankful for a fine surgical job, good medical care and rehabilitation; these are often forgotten in the ambition to profit from an industrial injury to the fullest extent.*

In spite of well-equipped modern factories, safety laws, safety programs, and improved health standards, industrial injuries remain a common occurence. Being injured, if unwisely encouraged, can become a most profitable industry.

Governments try to be fair, but making a "just society" is no easy matter. In 1964, Britain set up the Criminal Injuries Compensation Board to award financial compensation to the victims of crimes of violence. These unfortunate victims now spend much of their time sitting in their doctors' offices.

An Englishman injured in a train crash caused by an obstruction maliciously placed on the tracks can claim compensation from the board; if the train crashes because a wheel falls off, he cannot. If he is burned in a fire started by an arsonist, he can make a claim; but if the fire is started by a short circuit, he cannot. A good English father who cracks his head on his own bedroom door cannot make a claim; but an English lothario who seduces his neighbor's wife and gets punched in the face by her husband can make a claim. Such are the vagaries of the law. It seems difficult to believe that this really leads to more justice, but it certainly leads to more ill health.

It Takes Two to Tango

Some girls rape easily, and some people constantly end up by being victims. The new study of victimology seeks to delineate the character traits of these habitual victims. It usually takes two to make a victim, and the victim is often no passive partner. In some ways, it is no more sensible to reward victims for the results of their untoward behavior than it would be to reward gangsters for the perpetration of their crimes. Such arbitrary compensation just makes DOLP.

Accidents seldom just happen. It has been estimated that 88 percent of industrial accidents are not due to defective machinery or to dangerous conditions, but to the personality of the injured person. Relatively small numbers of people have relatively large numbers of accidents. Persons hospitalized with fractures may average four times as many accidents in their lives as patients admitted to hospitals with heart disease.

Laws for the compensation of personal injury too often hold one person responsible for what, in fact, are the defects of another's personality.

Compensation will not be useful until four conditions are met:

1. *The blame for an accident is fairly proportioned.*
2. *The claimant's disability is assessed only on the objective findings of the examining physicians.*
3. *This assessment is made against the background of the claimant's previous health.*
4. *Proper account is taken of the seriousness with which the claimant cooperated in the work of his rehabilitation.*

The present legal codes for compensation provide financial incentives for the injured litigant to remain unwell, and he usually does. Somebody else pays for his unnecessary illness.

Socially aware doctors all over the world have pointed out the disastrous effects on health of paying people large sums of money to be sick. Excellent reviews have been written of the medical studies made of compensation neurosis. Nearly 40 years ago, Dr. James Huddleson, in his study of the effects on health of compensation, warned:

> *Social custom and public opinion tend further to encourage the development of traumatic neurosis by their attitude toward the question of responsibility. The owner, the superior executive, some ulterior man-higher-up has become invariably chargeable, whether by law or by popular imagination, with final responsibility. The grocer's boy may drive as recklessly as he pleases, but let an accident occur and the responsibility is immediately an employer's. All the injured parties, including the reckless driver, can hope to be indemnified by the employer. Over against this scheme's advantages to the public must be set the growing feeling among all classes that responsibility can always be shifted from the individuals directly involved, to higher authority.*
>
> *If this is so, that responsibility can be passed*

along, then the recovery from a neurosis, instead of being the business of the person who exhibits it and for whose temporary benefit it has evolved, is the business of the employer or of the public, who may have no better approach to the problem than by indemnification. Those that have incentives for retaining a neurosis are not easy subjects for medical treatment; in fact, they can readily refuse treatment or practically nullify it by an attitude of demanding indemnity regardless of all else. The greater the sociological tendency towards this shifting of responsibility, the more frequent and the more refractory will traumatic neurosis become.

Dr. Huddleson uses the old term traumatic neurosis for what is now called compensation neurosis. Once doctors believed that it was the injury or trauma itself that produced the neurosis. But compensation claiming is now in fashion; and it has become clear that it is not the injury, but the possibility of financial reward, that produces the accompanying neurosis. Injuries acquired on the sports field get better faster than those acquired at work.

Recovery Lag

Compensation claiming delays recovery. When injured persons have been paired by the equal severity of their injuries, those who were claiming compensation have been found to recover far less quickly than those who were not. Of 500 patients who received treatment for comparable low back injuries in a hospital physiotheraphy department, half were eligible for compensation and half were not. Only 56 percent of the patients claiming compensation had improved enough to be discharged by the time 88 percent of the non-compensated group had been released. The compensation group of patients also received a significantly greater number of treatments.

Severity of the compensation neurosis is generally inversely proportionate to the severity of the accident or to its physical consequences: the less severe the injury, the more severe the compensation neurosis.

This is not surprising. If a man loses his legs and an arm in an industrial accident, no one will quibble about his need for compensation. He can try his hardest to make the best of a bad situation, and he will still get paid compensation. But if a man only loses a toe nail, then his claim for large financial compensation may be queried. His symptoms will need careful nurture and embellishment. His toe, he will claim, makes his whole leg ache so that he cannot walk properly. He has been so frightened by the accident that he cannot go near a machine again. The memory of it gives him nightmares so that he cannot sleep. He feels so exhausted he cannot do anything at all. He has no future. He has compensation neurosis.

Being run over by a bus or being mugged are the unfortunate hazards of life in the 20th century, just as being spiked by a rhinoceros or being bitten by a snake were natural hazards to our cave-dwelling ancestors. We live, or would like to live, in a caring society. Rather than fritter away our available resources on arbitrary compensation, it might be better if we supplied proper rehabilitation and adequate financial support to the victims of all accidents no matter how the accidents are caused.

Many victims would undoubtedly recover more quickly if this financial support were given in the form of wages paid for active cooperation and regular attendance at a rehabilitation center. When patients are paid for being sick rather than for getting well, both they and the rehabilitation staff become demoralized. The patients stay sick, and the rehabilitation staff gets fed up.

Doctor vs. Patient

As medicine becomes more impersonal, the hostility between patients and doctors increases. Some doctors leaven the monotony of clinical care by acquiring ever more expensive equipment, and by engaging in research. Such doctors turn their patients into guinea pigs. Some patients, distressed by their illness, lay the blame for everything upon their doctors.

We are—all of us—natural blame shifters, though some of us are more adept at it than others. One of the most adept is the writer of a letter to the *Toronto Star:*

> *While driving my car I was in collision with a deer on the highway. The collision killed the deer and did $300 damage to my car. I think someone should pay as it wasn't my fault, but the Lands and Forests Department says it's just one of those things. Who's responsible?*

If he was hospitalized, the answer is simple: the responsibility was his doctor's and the hospital's.

Blame shifting and compensation claiming can easily become a way of life. In California, enthusiasm for suing hospitals and doctors has reached epidemic proportions. Individual claims of over 1 million dollars against doctors are rocketing the costs of the insurance physicians must carry to protect themselves. A doctor in a high-risk specialty who has a record of a previous claim against him may now be paying as much as $16,000 in premiums. In spite of these high premiums, many American insurance companies are refusing to provide coverage for doctors. The companies claim they are losing too much money.

According to the law, an accident victim can sue a doctor who stopped to help, claiming that the help given was inadequate. Awards from this type of claim skyrocketed, and medical associations have therefore advised doctors against stopping at the scene of an accident to offer help. To encourage doctors to offer help to highway victims, many states have recently passed "good Samaritan laws" which protect public-spirited doctors against such claims.

Once blame shifting and compensation becomes a way of

life, habit and vested interests keep the system going. It is easy to encourage patients to be constantly on the take. Hospitals and doctors, by the nature of their work, will inevitably continue to provide ample opportunities for claims of malpractice. Nowadays, hospitals are devoting increasing amounts of their resources to protecting themselves against litigation. All sorts of expensive X-rays and other investigations are made —not for the patient's good—but for the protection of the hospital.

Since damage claiming has become an established practice, the cost of providing medical care has increased. Perhaps the constant threat of litigation makes doctors and hospitals more careful; but the situation also makes the physician and the hospital dislike their patients. In the long run this state of affairs will not be good for general health.

Sickness and Industry

Life in a modern industrial society is expensive. Many people require some kind of financial assistance when they are ill. In the United States, people usually have arrangements either with their employers or with private insurance companies to help pay for such emergencies. In Britain and other European countries, sickness benefits are provided by the state.

Much work time is lost through illness. There is always vocal concern for the 3 million working days that are lost each year in Britain through strikes, but 100 times this number of days are lost through sickness. In England, the average man loses 15 days per year for illness; women lose more.

The British do not take more time off to be sick than other Europeans. By contrast, American workers are either more conscientious or more healthy. In 1966, the average absence in the United States for illness was less than six days a year. In the last few years, this rate has gone up. One American expert writes rather anxiously:

*It is distinctly disturbing to think that, in time, the
absence rate in this country may approach and equal
those prevalent in certain European countries—double those we have experienced to date.*

It is probably inevitable that at the present stage of industrial development, work for most people has become
dreary and unrewarding. Perhaps quite reasonably many
workers are no longer prepared to work when they feel poor
with a cold. But health insurance schemes demand a doctor's
certificate before a sickness claim can be paid, and this puts
the doctor in a difficult position. No one can tell how sick
another person is feeling. The doctor signs the certificate; but
by doing so he often only endorses not his own opinion—but
his patient's opinion that he, the employee, is too sick to
work.

In Britain, most of the 10 million yearly claims for sickness benefits are for upper respiratory tract infections—for
colds, pharyngitis, viral bronchitis, and flu. There is no effective treatment for these virus diseases. Recovery occurs spontaneously within a few days, and the doctor has little useful
to offer for these conditions. His patients require his certificates, but not his skill.

Doctors Build Empires

A phony disease on a medical certificate which gains the worker
a few days free time with pay may have its uses, but should
doctors be encouraged to manufacture diseases? The medical
profession has an almost incorrigible habit of doing so. Like
other professionals, doctors seek to expand their territory.
Doctors deal in treatments, and treatments need diseases. It
was, for instance, an anonymous quack who, in promoting the
sale of his secret remedy at a half a sovereign a box, published *Ononia or the Heinous Sin of Self-Pollution;* and for
the next 250 years established masturbation as an important
and frequent cause of insanity. Dr. Henry Maudsley, as we

have seen, was one of his many respectable disciples.

Treatments of doubtful efficacy still help to define diseases. Doctors are not good at curing drunks, yet the World Health Organization defines alcoholism as follows:

> *Alcoholics are those excessive drinkers whose dependence on alcohol has attained such a degree that they show a noticeable mental disturbance or an interference with their mental and bodily health, their interpersonal relations and their smooth social and economic functioning; or who show the prodromal signs of such developments. They therefore require treatment.*

Supplying treatment for all these alcoholics may not do them much good, but supplying treatment will certainly provide jobs for psychiatrists.

Nor does the psychiatrist's lack of success in treating alcoholics inhibit the Committee on Alcoholism of the WHO from commenting that

> *In many countries, adult males in need of treatment for alcoholism outnumber those in need for tuberculosis by several hundred percent.*

In 1965, the American Psychiatric Association issued an edict that psychiatrists and other physicians should extend to alcoholics the same care afforded to other ill people. Approximately 5 million alcoholic Americans were admitted to the nest of sickness and tucked safely and profitably under the doctor's wing.

Doctors do not have much success with curing alcoholics, but they have absolutely none with curing psychopaths. Perhaps the most salient characteristic of the psychopath is that, in spite of all medical and legal intervention, his behavior remains as boisterously anti-social as ever. Such treatment failure did not, however, deter the authors of the 1959 British

Mental Health Act from using the psychopath's need for treatment in defining this condition:

> *In this Act "psychopathic disorder" means a persistent disorder or disability of the mind which results in abnormally aggressive or seriously irresponsible conduct on the part of the patient, and requires or is susceptible to medical treatment.*

Certainly the law has little that is constructive to offer in the curtailment of the undesirable behavior of the alcoholic and the psychopath. But then again, neither has the medical profession. By pretending he has a solution to these problems up his sleeve, a doctor just makes it more difficult for society to find other and perhaps more useful means of managing socially destructive conduct.

Medical Paternalism

It is, of course, no new thing for doctors to turn behavior they disapprove of into illness. Such a metamorphosis also turns the doctor into somebody with the authority to do something about it. Let me give an historical example: Dr. Samuel A. Cartwright in his "Report on the Disease and Physical Peculiarities of the Negro Race," published in 1851 in the then prestigious *New Orleans Medical and Surgical Journal,* described the new disease of drapetomania. Dr. Cartwright named this disease from *drapetes,* meaning a runaway slave, and *mania* meaning madness. He wrote:

> *In noticing a disease not heretofore classed among the long list of maladies that man is subject to, it was necessary to have a new term to express it. The cause, in the most of cases, that induces the negro to run away from service, is as much a disease of the mind as any other species of mental alienation, and much more curable, as a general rule. With the ad-*

*vantages of proper medical advice, strictly followed,
this troublesome practice that many negroes have of
running away, can be almost entirely prevented, although the slaves be located on the borders of a free
State, within a stone's throw of the abolitionists. . . .*

Treatment of drapetomania consisted of punishing the
runaway slaves until they returned to that submissive state
which God had intended for them.

*They then only had to be kept in that state, and
treated like children with care, kindness, attention
and humanity, to prevent and cure them from running away. . . .*

Medical paternalism has not abated. "The long list of
maladies that man is subject to" has been substantially length-
ened since Dr. Cartwright's day. Worries and misery now
are also disorders of the mind amenable to medical attention.
The middle-aged woman who steals from Woolworth's is unwell; the heroin addict sick. A rich and varied sex life may no
longer land us in court, but it often leads us to the doctor.
Few are left who have not at some time been labeled sick,
and unable to manage without a doctor's fatherly care. This
certainly increases the size of the medical empire; but it is
doubtful if it reduces the totality of our unhappiness, or that
it makes our behavior any more satisfactory.

Certainly those of us who are making a miserable mess of
our lives can, if we so choose, sometimes use professional help
to find a more satisfactory way of living. But by accepting
uncomfortable adjustment and unsatisfactory behavior as illness, doctors often end up by extending to us the right to
continue as we are. It is axiomatic in modern society that no
one can help being sick. But doctors, if they are to be useful, should not make more illness than is necessary.

Neither should society make illness a necessity. If we
make sickness the only way of survival, or even the only way

to acquire a comfortable life, then people will be sick. In the low employment years after World War I, many British veterans could support themselves and their families only by remaining on the sick list. A noted healer who was reputed to cure all ailments paid a visit to some of these soldiers. They were so frightened at the prospect of certain cure that one after the other was seized with convulsions. The healer retired in confusion.

Modern welfare states are being created to abolish the kind of society in which a man must be sick to be fed. But this is certainly easier talked about than done. Our resources, both human and financial, are limited.

We can give either small amounts of help to everybody or large amounts to a few. If we give small amounts of help to everyone, we waste it upon the affluent and competent, and provide insufficiently for the needy. If we restrict help to those in want, we seduce more people into being needy, in order to obtain such help. This is the dilemma in which all welfare states are now finding themselves. Help often backfires.

SOURCES

Adler, A.: "The Psychology of Repeated Accidents in Industry." *American Journal of Psychiatry,* **122** 454 (1965).

Annual Conference of Representatives of Local Medical Committees: National Insurance Certification. *British Medical Journal Supplements,* **2** 156 (1967); **2** 155 (1969); **2** 179 (1970).

Brain, W. R.: "After Injuries to the Central Nervous System." In "Discussion on Rehabilitation." *Proceedings of the Royal Society of Medicine,* **35** 302 (1942).

Crawley, Jerry: "The Lamentations of a Jeremiah." *Industrial Medicine and Surgery,* **36** 394 (1967).

Criminal Injuries Compensation Board: *Fourth Report.* London: Her Majesty's Stationery Office, 1968.

Department of Health and Social Security: *Annual Report for the Year 1970.* London: Her Majesty's Stationery Office, 1971.

Dukar, B.: "Die psychogenen Reaktionen in der Versicherungs Medizin." *Schwizerische Medizinische Wochenschrift,* **80** 405, 479 (1950).

Dunbar, F.: "Medical Aspects of Accidents and Mistakes in the Industrial Army and Armed Forces." *War Medicine,* **4** 161 (1943).

Feber, Stanley, and Sheriden, Bart: "Who'll Stop Runaway Malpractice Insurance Rates?" *Medical Economics,* **47** (12) 230 (1970).

Fetterman, J. L.: "Neuropsychiatric Aspects of Industrial Accidents." *Industrial Medicine and Surgery,* **15** 96 (1946).

Freund, Paul A.: *Experimentation with Human Subjects.* London: George Allen and Unwin, 1972.

Glyn, John: "Some Factors Influencing the Duration of Morbidity in Industry." *Proceedings of the Royal Society of Medicine,* **63** 1131 (1970).

Great Britain: Mental Health Act 1951; Section 4 (4).

Hare, E. M.: "Masturbation Insanity: The History of an Idea." *Journal of Mental Science,* **108** 1 (1962).

Hirschfeld, A. H.: "The Accident Process: An Overview." *Journal of Rehabilitation,* 33 27 (1967).

Huddleson, James H.: *Accidents, Neurosis and Compensation.* Baltimore: Williams and Wilkins Co., 1932.

Kennedy, F.: "Mind of the Injured Worker: Its Effect upon Disability Periods." *Compensation Medicine,* 1 19 (1946).

Krusen, E. M., and Ford, D. E.: "Compensation Factor in Low Back Injury." *Journal of the American Medical Association,* **166** 1128 (1958).

Medical World News: "Malpractice." **10** (43) 34 (1969).

Ong, John R.: "Some Paradoxes of Workman's Compensation." *Industrial Medicine and Surgery,* **36** 468 (1967).

Pappworth, M. H.: *Human Guinea Pigs: Experimentation on Man.* London: Routledge and Kegan Paul, 1967.

Pokorny, A. D., and Moore, F. J.: "Neurosis and Compensation." *Archives of Industrial Hygiene and Occupational Medicine,* **8** 547 (1953).

Rawson, A. J.: "Accident Proneness." *Psychosomatic Medicine,* **6** 88 (1944).

Smith, David J.: "Absenteeism and 'Presenteeism' in Industry." *Archives of Environmental Health,* **21** 670 (1970).

Szasz, Thomas S.: "The Sane Slave: An Historical Note on the Use of Medical Diagnosis as Justificatory Rhetoric." *American Journal of Psychotherapy,* **24** 228 (1971).

Time: "Is the Victim Guilty?" (Canadian Edition), July 5, 1971.

U.S. Department of Health, Education and Welfare, Public Health Service: *Disability Days in the United States July 1965–June 1966.* (Publication 1000).
———: *Vital and Health Statistics: National Center for Health Statistics* (Washington), Series 10, No. 47, 1968.

White, T. H.: *The Age of Scandal.* London: Jonathan Cape, 1950.

Wootton, Barbara: *Social Science and Social Pathology.* London: George Allen and Unwin, 1959.

World Health Organization Expert Committee on Mental Health: *Alcohol Subcommittee Second Report. WHO Technical Report Series No. 48* (1952).

Life in the
Mental Hospitals

The whole earth is our hospital
Endowered by a ruined millionaire
Wherein if we do well, we shall
Die of that absolute paternal care
That will not leave us, but prevents us everywhere.

T. S. ELIOT

A proverb says: "Do not remove a fly from your neighbor's forehead with a hatchet." Yes, help is a dubious commodity.

There is, of course, nothing dubious about helping your wife with household chores, if you both work. But if you keep her at home and do everything for her—supply her with servants, shop for her, protect her from worries, and give her lollipops when she cries—she will, after a few years of such treatment, be as competent as a three-year-old. Such help is not useful.

Humans differ from all other species of mammals by the many years it takes to become fully grown—that is, to become adult. During the long period of our immaturity, we are dependent upon parental care. If we are to survive childhood, we need the help of adults. Any child wields enormous power, for his very helplessness forces others to care for him. When a four-year-old runs out of the front door onto a busy road for the tenth time in one afternoon, he knows he can still make somebody chase out after him and bring him back to safety.

153

"Baby Help"

Some of us as we grow up are reluctant to surrender this delicious power. Childish behavior in the adult continues to command attention. A 40-year-old woman who for the tenth time swallows an overdose of barbiturates knows that the doctor will still have to wash out her stomach, however reluctant he is to do so. The help that is the baby's birthright, but which is demanded by adults from other adults, I will call—for want of a more formal name—"Baby Help."

Unlike mutual help, both the giving and the demanding of Baby Help is coercive. Portnoy's mom forces the last spoonful down a retching throat; the spoiled man throws a temper tantrum because his wife will not help him find his shoes. As society becomes polarized into the helpers and the helpless, Baby Help is often the coinage of their interaction.

Stimulated by the social chaos of World War II, men became more interested in social groups, in how groups of people live and interact. This new breed of scientists—the sociologists—found the small world of the mental hospitals a convenient locale for their studies.

Studies soon revealed the disastrous effects that mental hospitals were having upon their patients. Here are seen the worst effects of help. The results of Baby Help can be most clearly demonstrated. Lessons learned in these hospitals have application far beyond the confines of their gray walls.

Those who are unlucky enough to be admitted to a mental hospital go there either because their brains are not working properly, or because they have not learned to cope adequately with the demands life puts upon us all. In either case, such patients are extremely vulnerable to social collapse, and to letting other people look after them.

Mental hospitals are veritable factories of dependency. They absolutely insure that those who tenant them do not take care of themselves.

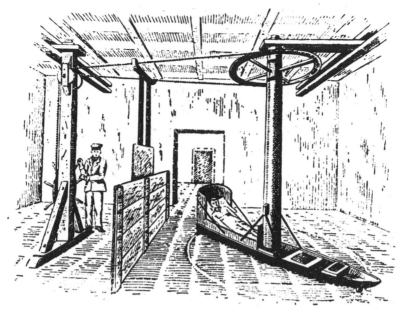

The whirling bed treatment.

The gyrating chair treatment.

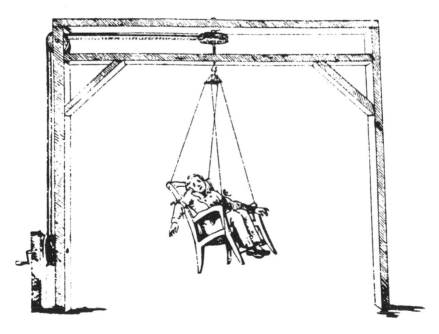

Curing Insanity with Discomfort

Mental hospitals have always been rather nasty places. On the supposition that physical discomfort, illness, and mental illness are mutually exclusive, Erasmus Darwin, grandfather of the famed Charles Darwin, introduced whirling treatments into psychiatry. Strapped into a spinning bed, a patient was whirled until blood oozed from his mouth, his ears, or his nose. Benjamin Rush lost no time in importing this treatment into the U.S., and with his gyrating chair he soon had the American insane on the spin. Rush also advocated large bleedings for his patients. In his day, he was known as "the lancet-loving physician of Philadelphia." He is now known as the father of American psychiatry, and it is his head that appears on the medallion of the American Psychiatric Association.

The "hollow wheel" and the "cold water douche" treatment were also popular treatments for the insane in the last century. They were convenient ways of giving nasty shocks to obstreperous patients and, as with all treatments, remarkable cures were attributed to them. Patients can be exceedingly aggravating, and "compulsory helpers" soon feel vindictive. Such treatments must certainly have made the staff of mental hospitals feel better.

Such is the nature of help and treatment that many of the advances in the management of the mentally ill have been made not by the introduction of new treatment—but by the discarding of old ones.

The Method of Non-Restraint

The first big improvement in institutional environment came at the end of the 18th century when Philippe Pinel, in Paris, showed that lunatics did not have to be chained up for their own or for anyone else's protection. It was Rush who removed the chains from the American insane, but Rush, like many present day psychiatrists, believed in tranquilization. He popularized his tranquilizing chair, which restrained a patient's

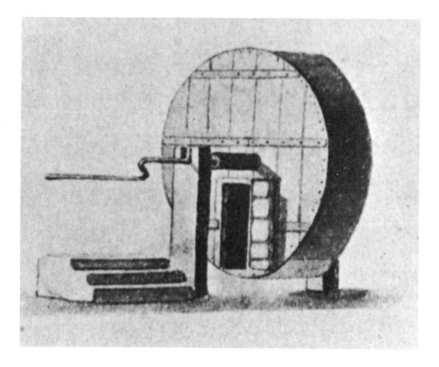

The hollow wheel treatment.

every movement as well as restricting his vision. The next improvement happened in the early 1840s at Hanwell Hospital (now St. Bernard's) in London when John Conolly untied the patients and once more demonstrated that lunatics do not have to be treated like wild animals. What became known as the English system of non-restraint spread throughout the world.

The United States was an exception. Certainly Conolly's non-restraint regime was well known; it was discussed at nearly every meeting of the American Association of Medical Superintendents for the next 50 years. But the hospital superintendents did not like Conolly's methods. They even regarded these new-fangled notions as downright unpatriotic:

The patients in European institutions, accustomed as they were to unquestioned acceptance of authority, might willingly submit to "moral restraint," but not your liberty-loving American, who sane or insane, would never agree placidly to the imposition of authority by an individual, and hence could be restrained only by mechanical means.

Employing the Patients

In Canada, Conolly's non-restraint approach met with a kinder reception. Dr. Richard Bucke, a pioneer Canadian psychia-

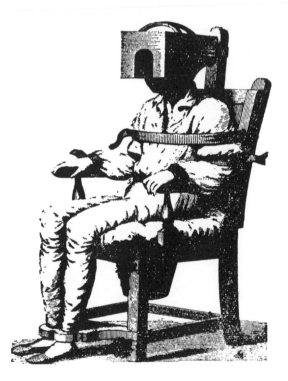

Benjamin Rush's tranquilizing chair.

trist, admired Conolly's ideas and introduced them into his hospital at London, Ontario. Bucke removed all forms of mechanical restraint from his patients, and he also insisted that his patients shouldn't be drugged nor be drunk. He argued that alcohol had no place in the treatment of insanity. Bucke provided nearly all his patients with some kind of meaningful employment. In his annual report in 1884, he wrote:

During the year just closed and for three months before that—that is during the last fifteen months—we have not used at this Asylum any mechanical restraint or seclusion of any kind whatever; neither have we during that time used any morphia, chloral, or other sedative drug for the purpose of quieting or calming any noisy or violent patient. Two years ago, we began in earnest this non-restraint movement, and I must confess I have been as much surprised as any one else can be at the success we have had in carrying it out. It is not simply that we have disused mechanical restraint and seclusion, but we have revolutionized at the same time the whole morale of the institution, the disuse of restraint and seclusion being only a small part of the revolution. The central element in the change to which I refer is undoubtedly the employment of the patients. It is this far more than anything else that has enabled us to do without restraint.

Although mental hospitals everywhere continued to be built a long way from cities and were surrounded by high walls, they did offer a more dignified asylum to those people whose odd behavior made them unacceptable to the outside world. Asylums all over the world soon had their own farms and market gardens, and staff and patients worked in these gardens together. Many of their nursing staffs were also trained tradesmen. Furniture, clothes, shoes, and other hospital requirements were made and repaired by staff and pa-

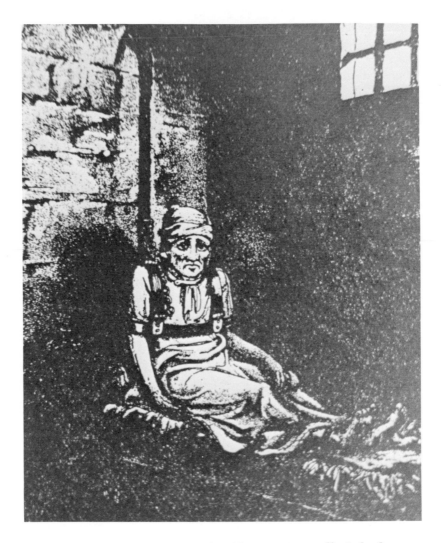

James Norris was in irons for 10 years in a cell of the lower gallery at Bethlam Hospital, London. The wall-and-chain apparatus was one of many forms of mechanical restraint of the insane.

tients in large hospital workshops. Patients were provided with man-sized employment, and they could remain useful and productive members of their small communities.

"Curing" Mental Illness

But doctors have the treatment bug. In World War II, psychiatry proved itself useful; and in doing so, its practitioners developed megalomania. Mental illness, psychiatrists claimed, could be cured. Attention became devoted to treatment: to shock treatment, to lobotomy, and to insulin coma. Farms and gardens were sold off to help pay for the rising costs of these treatments, and the hospital workshops were closed down. More domestic and maintenance staff were employed to do the ordinary everyday work that had previously been done by patients, who were now to devote their full time to being cured.

In spite of the new treatment, the mental hospitals remained full, but their patients were no longer provided with anything to do. They sat about in drab wards or wandered aimlessly down long corridors. Today, in many mental hospitals, they continue to do just this. Often patients cannot even keep their own wards clean, because working patients threaten to reduce hospital jobs and the unions don't like that. A cobbler must stick to his last; and a patient must only do his own job, which is *to be looked after.*

Inducing Apathy

Modern psychiatry with its emphasis on treatment has managed to destroy much that was useful in the old asylums.

Absence of occupation is not rest;
A mind quite vacant is a mind distress'd.

So sang the poet Cowper. Dr. Russell Barton, the psychiatrist, said the same thing in prose. In 1959, before he quit

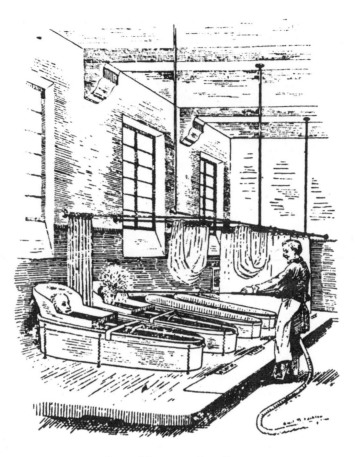

The cold-water douche treatment.

England for America, Dr. Barton introduced the now inter-
nationally known term "institutional neurosis" to describe the
lethargy that enslaves the patients in a mental hospital.

Added to the effects of their original illnesses are those
of enforced idleness and apathy-producing drugs. Dr. Barton's description of this condition is graphic:

> *Institutional neurosis is a disease characterized by*
> *apathy, lack of initiative, loss of interest (more*

marked in things and events not immediately pres-
ent), submissiveness, and sometimes no expression of
feelings of resentment at harsh or unfair orders.
There is a lack of interest in the future, and an ap-
parent inability to make practical plans for it, a
deterioration in personal habits, toilet, and standards
generally, a loss of individuality, and a resigned ac-
ceptance that things will go on as they are—unchang-
ingly, inevitably, and indefinitely.

Dr. Conolly taught that mechanical restraint of mentally
ill patients equals neglect. People can also be kept docile by
drugs. Dr. Conolly's son-in-law, the famous Dr. Maudsley,
was vigorously opposed to such use of drugs. "We make,"
wrote Maudsley, "a solitude and call it peace."

Dr. Conolly had used the term mechanical restraint, and
Dr. Maudsley introduced the term "chemical restraint" to
describe the growing habit of controlling behavior by the
stupefying action of drugs. He wrote:

Although the mischief still goes on, especially in pri-
vate practice, in two or three large public asylums,
each containing more than a thousand inmates, it has
been found practical almost entirely to abandon the
use of them.

Yet, 75 years later, Dr. Barton was writing about a similar misuse of drugs:

It is not surprising that the majority of patients forced
to go to bed by 7:00 P.M. after an idle day require
sedatives to sleep, nor that they wake after 8 hours
at 3 or 4 A.M. (or are awakened by the clanking
keys or noise caused by the rounds nurse who may
shine a torch at them) and require more sedatives for
further sleep. If, as sometimes happens, this be given
at 4:00 A.M. the patient may be difficult to awaken

at 6:00 A.M. and not in a very fit state to have her bed made, complete her toilet, and help with breakfast. The effect of the sedative may not wear off from 4 to 12 hours after it is given, so that during the morning the apathy produced by the absence of a planned routine and loss of contact with the world outside the hospital is furthered by the effects of paraldehyde, barbituric acid derivatives, or the modern tranquilizing drugs, chlorpromazine and reserpine.

During the day paraldehyde or barbiturates have been favorite remedies for "disturbed behavior." Other patients may be having regular sedation with paraldehyde, barbituric acid derivatives, reserpine, or phenothiazines, some of which not only predispose to apathy but may cause addiction which binds the patient to the mental hospital even more strongly, and makes the idea of discharge repugnant.

Drugging often starts with the admission ward. The nurse may almost routinely ask for the patient to have 6 gr. of sodium amytal or 2 oz. of haustus paraldehyde.

Stopping treatment often turns out to be the best treatment. Dr. Barton found that "distranquilization," as soon as the principle was accepted by his hospital staff, often produced gratifying results.

When we insist on putting together large numbers of not very resourceful people and requesting from them no form of constructive or responsible behavior, then boredom alone insures their petulant and difficult behavior. We no longer train our nurses to be builders, farmers, gardeners, typists, factory workers, or cooks so that they can aid a psychiatric patient in his process of rehabilitation; indeed, such activities are now considered alien to the professional status of a nurse.

Today's nurses are seldom permitted or able to participate with their patients in any form of learning or constructive behavior. When we teach our nurses only how to treat illness

—to hand out pills and give injections—that is what they will do. Nurses will stay nurses, and patients will stay patients.

Under the inspiration of a handful of enlightened doctors, some changes to the better have gradually been made in the way of life in mental hospitals. Patients are being given more freedom, more work, and more responsibility. These changes seem to be proving useful. Similar changes in the treatment of the chronically sick outside hospitals might be equally effective.

The Open Door Policy

Dingleton Hospital, a small mental hospital 37 miles south of Edinburgh, Scotland, won for itself international renown as the first mental hospital to give its patients more freedom. In 1949, Dr. George Bell, its superintendent, opened all the locked wards and removed the bars from the windows. He thus initiated the "open door policy" which, like Conolly's non-restraint movement before it, soon spread through Britain and to other countries, as well.

When patients are confined in locked wards, they are presented with the challenge to escape, and often spend much of their time trying to do so. When the doors were opened, it was discovered that few patients actually wanted to leave. They preferred the security of the hospital; they liked being looked after.

It has become clear that it is far easier to keep most patients in hospitals than it is to keep them out of the hospital. The open door has turned into a revolving one. Discharged patients are often only too keen on coming back again.

St. Lawrence State Hospital in New York State was the first United States mental hospital to adopt an open door policy. Superintendent Herman B. Snow described an incident that happened shortly after his long-stay wards were opened: a patient came back to the ward leading his injured friend by the hand. They had heard a noise in the sky, and although they had heard the sound of airplanes before from their locked ward, they had never been able to see an aircraft. They had become so excited at seeing an airplane for the first time that they forgot to look where they were going, and one of the patients fell down.

In such protective ways, mental hospitals were supposed to be helping their patients to recover and to face life in the 20th century! Only very few patients need to be treated with such sheltered care. Dr. Snow, like the other superintendents who opened their wards, found that when patients were given their freedom, they act much the same as other people. Certainly, there are some exceptions; but on the whole, mental hospital patients do not hurt either themselves or hurt other people. They are no more dangerous than the rest of us. Medical paternalism is not useful.

Doctors like to claim that their treatments are useful. It is often said that it was the introduction of the new tranquilizing drugs that made the open door policy possible. Possibly. But Dr. Bell had successfully opened the last of his ward doors three years before chlorpromazine was introduced into psychiatric practice.

Work Therapy

It is hardly surprising that it was the industrious Germans who first introduced work therapy into modern psychiatry, but they did not continue this program for long. Handicapped and dependent people are vulnerable. Hitler sent the patients in German mental hospitals to the gas chambers.

The equally industrious neighbors of the Germans, the Dutch, continued with work therapy. For nearly half a century, their mental hospitals have demonstrated how much useful work even severely handicapped people can do; and how much the provision of a meaningful occupation prevents the personality deterioration that, in other parts of the world, is considered to be an integral part of mental illness. Patients are expected not only to do many of the maintenance jobs in their hospitals—but also to help pay for the cost of hospital upkeep by the manufacture of clothes, footwear, and other goods for commercial sale.

In English and American mental hospitals, where meaningful work was no longer being provided, attempts were made to provide other activities. Occupational therapists were employed to teach pottery, weaving, and basketmaking. These activities did not prove to be a success.

Industrial therapy, though not a panacea, is proving more useful. Workshops are established in hospitals, and contracts are made with local factories, which then send in work to be done by the patients in the workshops. Paying patients for the work they do provides an effective incentive for many to start some kind of structured activity again.

Such workshops have not been easy to establish. Mental hospitals, in Britain, Canada, and the United States, are government-run; and while governments seem prepared to provide unending funds for pills—because pills are treatment and therefore special—these same governments are not so willing to provide funds for workshops.

This is a short-sighted policy. Not only do hospitals with good workshops rehabilitate their patients more successfully than hospitals without them, but the program saves the government money.

Richard Bucke and others demonstrated a hundred years ago that, when patients are provided with proper employment, their need for sedative drugs is much reduced. Patients in the 20th century are no different. Those hospitals with established vigorous work and retraining programs have a smaller drug bill than do those that allow their patients to sit around all day and do nothing. Since mental hospitals have huge drug bills, the savings in drugs alone would go a long way toward paying for the establishment and the maintenance of the workshops.

Persuading often reluctant patients to swallow pills four times a day is costly of hospital staff time. For a mental hospital of average size, it has been estimated that the distribution of medication to the patients takes 93 nursing hours a day. This equals the work of 15 full-time nurses. This number of hospital staff could run a large workshop.

In one British mental hospital in which I worked, an enthusiastic head gardener was probably responsible for the recovery of more patients than any of the medical or nursing staff. All the patients who could go to his garden he set to work on potting plants, grafting roses, and growing vegetables. The patients were delighted to discover their own green fingers. When attention is paid to success and not to sickness, patients get better.

Sadly, doctors, nurses, and health bureaucracies nearly always find it easier to provide for sickness rather than for health. In 1971, the British Government moved responsibility for the care of retarded children from the Department of Health to the Ministry of Education. Doctors and nurses were teaching retarded children how to swallow pills and how to be patients. They were not teaching them any social skills.

Mental hospitals on both sides of the Atlantic have had varying success in providing meaningful occupations for their patients. Some have developed workshops profitable enough to support their total cost. Enough incentive pay is provided so that patients are pleased to work in these workshops.

Unfortunately, such success is limited to a few hospitals. In most cases, industrial therapy work is no more high grade than the fixing together of the parts of plastic toys. Many hospitals do not cater to more than a handful of their patients.

In defense of mental hospitals, it must be said that many of the people who drift in and out of them have, over the years, become dependent for their keep upon the state. Since these patients usually intend to go on being so, it is unrealistic both for them to accept work training, and for hospitals to provide them with work retraining programs. These dependent patients are usually the ones who stay sick. Interestingly, Philippe Pinel after he had released the Parisian insane from their chains and provided them with a variety of occupations, complained that "members of the nobility who reject such activities are especially difficult to cure."

The Therapeutic Community

The therapeutic community concept was originated in England, at the War Neurosis Unit of the Belmont Hospital in the late 1940s. The idea caught on, and now most mental hospitals on both sides of the Atlantic at least pretend to organize themselves along such lines.

A therapeutic community makes not only the doctor, but everybody, including the patients themselves, responsible for getting patients better. A therapeutic community aims to use everyone's skills, so that patients are no longer so dependent upon the sometimes rather limited capabilities of doctors.

Ward meetings of patients and staff are held regularly, and at these meetings the therapeutic goals of the community are discussed. Patients are held responsible, not only for participating in their own recovery, but for setting limits to each other's anti-social behavior. Patients are not allowed to sit back and wait indefinitely for somebody else to get them better.

Splints for the damaged mind are not useful. Although superficially the tradition of excusing a sick and suffering person from supporting himself or from being a participating member of a social group may be a humane one, such exemption from responsibility is often damaging. The social skills necessary to manage life outside a hospital are soon lost through disuse, and an "illness" soon becomes chronic and incurable. Excusing people from responsibility can become the opposite of the humane practice that it is intended to be.

Chronic sickness and other handicaps need not be barriers to success. Helen Keller was deaf and blind since two, but by hard work she learned to talk and turned her life into a success. Franklin D. Roosevelt, paralyzed from the waist down, became President of the world's most powerful nation. Handicapped employees who choose to work have less absenteeism and better records than do comparable groups of able-bodied workers.

It is more constructive, and indeed kinder, to expect from

those who are handicapped, physically or mentally, a more than average effort to succeed. Only then can the handicapped person avoid the added misfortune of personal failure.

Hospital or Hotel?

Mental hospitals have been aptly described as institutions without culture. For many who are tired of the struggle of living in the world and who are prepared to set low the sights of their ambition, hospital life can offer the comforts of a bland existence. Television and all other modern necessities are provided. The staff is usually friendly, and so far as general behavior is concerned, everything goes. Many of the big mental hospitals incorporate an adolescent unit, and so provide an unending supply of promiscuous girls.

Most large mental hospitals were built in the last century to provide for those ill-treated or neglected by their own communities. These buildings are old and drab; by present-day standards, their accommodations are abysmal. Governments are under constant pressure to do something about these antiquated institutions.

In 1963, faced with 800,000 Americans packed into the nation's mental institutions and a great deal of propaganda about the potential success of modern psychiatric treatments, President John Kennedy urged Congress to pass the Community Mental Health Act. This law established *community* mental health centers which were to provide modern psychiatric care for America's mentally sick.

The British government is going even further; it no longer plans to build any large mental hospitals. Many of the mentally ill will be transferred to smaller psychiatric hospitals and units.

Plans to provide alternative care for the mentally ill are quite proper, but they do present a problem both to the doctors and to the community. The old hospitals were pretty awful places; yet people wanted to stay in them. The new hospitals are much nicer, and not surprisingly, even more people want to stay in them. A report in the *British Journal of Psychiatry* on a year's experience at one such hospital, opened in 1967, states:

> *There was evidence that the comfort and convenience of the new hospital made it an attractive refuge from the troubles and unpleasantness of life. Patients, particularly those with social problems, sought to prolong their stay; discharge was postponed by hysterical manoeuvres, failure to survive trial in employment, or threats of suicide if forced to leave. Others outside, trading on a known psychiatric disability, tried to blackmail their way in. It became clear that certain patients knew the ropes and that requests for emergency admission tended to occur late at night or at the weekends, when the unsuspecting duty doctor might not be aware of the patients' previous record in the ward.*

Keeping patients out is a problem even at the old and forbidding hospital in which I work. A few months ago, we discovered that the local bar pinned up a weekly list of the days when the doctors of the hospital were on duty. A hospital's clientele soon learns which doctors are pushovers, and when it is worth a try to get in.

If it were possible to select only people with problems who might benefit from a stay in one of these new hospitals and to reject the rest, then these hospitals would be useful. But if doctors are allowed to select their own patients, they usually end up by choosing only nice middle-class patients who are not very ill.

When mental hospitals have to take more or less anyone who is either crazy or who by his odd behavior inconveniences the community, then many people are admitted against the better judgment of the staff. Such hospitals often have nothing useful to offer to many of its patients.

Also, a considerable number of people find that a mental

hospital is better than the most comfortable commercial hotel they can afford. Such a person manages to use the hospital as his hotel. This kind of misuse not only discourages the staff, but also costs the community a great deal of money. On either side of the Atlantic, the cost of supporting each patient in one of these new units is about two or three times the cost of an ordinary working man's wage.

Doctors and nurses know very well that hospital patients often abuse their services. But these professionals have chosen the role of the helper. Patients are by popular definition helpless, and therefore requiring of help. It is the hospital's duty to take care of a patient until he is better.

But what is being better? Have you, dear reader, ever tried to discharge an enthusiastic patient? He wanders into the nearest police station, threatens to shoot the President or

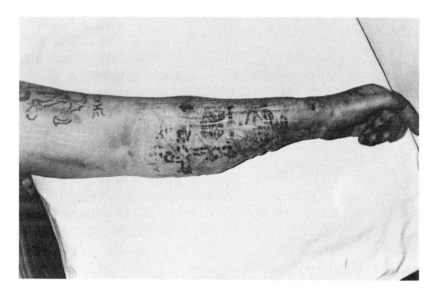

This is an arm of a man who has come to like being in mental hospitals. Each time he is discharged, he goes to some public place and slashes his arms with a razor. The police then bring him straight back to the hospital.

whispers the magic word *suicide*. He is then returned to the hospital, and the hospital is criticized for discharging the poor man in such a sorry state of mind. The patient gets another lesson in the usefulness of illness, and the doctor in the helplessness of the compulsory helper.

Is Mental Illness a Myth?

Dr. Thomas Szasz infuriates his colleagues by claiming persuasively that mental illness is a myth. He writes elegantly on the polarization of society into helpers and helpless:

> *Like the infant's cry, the message "I am sick" is exceedingly effective in mobilizing others to some kind of helpful action. In accordance with this communicative impact of sickness, physicians—following in the footsteps of their predecessors, the clergy—have tended to define their occupation as a "calling." This implied that it was not only the sick and helpless who were calling them, as indeed they were, but God as well. The helpers would thus hasten to the side of the helpless (the sick or disabled), and would minister to him to restore him to "health." This sort of therapeutic attitude tends to define the role of the helpless or sick person in a complimentary manner, that is, as entitled to help, merely by the virtue of being disabled. Hence, if we do not help him (particularly if we could), we incur moral blame for our failure.*
>
> *It frequently happens that this "game of helpfulness" is played so that those who are on the help-giving team have unknowingly obligated themselves to caring for the help-seekers. They no longer choose to offer or withhold help, depending on circumstances, but instead are committed to an unwritten social contract that may be quite burdensome for them.*

Dr. Szasz has emphasized that helpers—be they politicians, priests, physicians, or parents—"foster non-learning behavior." A parent may reward his child's persistent helplessness and dependency in order to enhance his (the father's or mother's) own importance and self-esteem. Dr. Szasz thunders:

> *This constitutes a significant part of the grand total of human tendencies that press towards childishness, helplessness, incompetence and "mental illness"!*

The lines appearing at the opening of this chapter are from "East Coker" in *Four Quartets*, copyright 1943 by T. S. Eliot; renewed 1971 by Esme Valerie Eliot. Reprinted by permission of Harcourt Brace Jovanovich, Inc.

SOURCES

Ackerknect, Erwin H.: *A Short History of Psychiatry*. New York: Hafner Publishing Co., 1959.

Barton, Russell: *Institutional Neurosis*. Bristol: John Wright & Son, 1959.

Bucke, Richard: *Annual Report for the Year 1884*. Ontario.

Caudhill, W. A.: *The Psychiatric Hospital as a Small Society*. Cambridge: Harvard University Press, 1958.

Clark, David H.: *Administrative Therapy*. London: Tavistock Publications, 1964.

Council on Occupational Health: "Employment of the Handicapped." *Journal of the American Medical Association,* **187** 234 (1964).

Department of Health Social Security: *Better Services for the Mentally Handicapped*. London: Her Majesty's Stationery Office, 1971.

Deutch, Albert: *The Mentally Ill in America*. New York: Columbia University Press, 1949.

Goffman, Erving: *Asylums*. New York: Anchor Books, Doubleday & Co., 1961.

Greenland, Cyril: "Three Pioneers of Canadian Psychiatry." *Journal of the American Medical Association,* **200** 833 (1967).

Haden, Philip: "Drugs—Single or Multiple Daily Dosage?" *American Journal of Psychiatry,* **115** 932 (1959).

Hunter, Richard, and MacAlpine, Ida: *Three Hundred Years of Psychiatry 1535–1860*. London: Oxford University Press, 1963.

Jones, Maxwell: "Intra and Extra Mural Community Psychiatry." *American Journal of Psychiatry,* **117** 784 (1961).

Kennedy, John F.: *Mental Illness and Mental Retardation*. Message to Congress, Feb. 5, 1963.

Kraepelin, Emit: "Hundert Jahre Psychiatrie." *Zeitschrift fur die gesampte Neurologie und Psychiatrie,* **38** 161 (1918).

Maudsley, Henry: *The Pathology of the Mind*. London: Macmillan, 1895.

Morison, Sir Alexander: *Cases of Mental Disease with Practical Observations.* London: Longman and Highley, 1828.

Rapoport, Robert N.: *Community as Doctor.* London: Social Sciences Paperbacks, 1960.

Roback, A. A., and Kierman, Thomas: *Pictorial History of Psychology and Psychiatry.* New York: Philosophical Library, 1969.

Snow, Herman B.: "Dingleton Hospital, Melrose." In "Impressions of Scottish Hospitals." *Journal of Hospital and Community Psychiatry.* (APA), **16** 253 (1965).

————: "The Open Door Hospital." *Canadian Journal of Public Health,* **49** 363 (1958).

Stanton, Alfred M., and Schwartz, Morris S.: *The Mental Hospital.* New York: Basic Books Inc., 1954.

Szasz, Thomas: *The Myth of Mental Illness.* New York: Dell Publishing Co., 1961.

Woodside, Moya: "Are Observation Wards Obsolete? A Review of One Year's Experience in an Acute Male Psychiatric Admission Unit." *British Journal of Psychiatry,* **114** 1013 (1968).

Zusman, Jack: "Sociology and Mental Illness: Some Neglected Implications for Treatment." *Archives of General Psychiatry,* **15** 635 (1966).

In Loco Parentis

When her kittens are small, a mother cat is completely attentive to their needs. She frets and fusses about them and is reluctant to leave them even for a minute. But as her kittens grow bigger, she becomes blasé. She suckles them only when she feels like it, and she is impervious to their mews for help. Only when a kitten is in serious trouble does she race to the rescue.

Eight-month-old baby baboons grow so heavy that their mothers refuse to carry them any longer. The babies do not like walking through the long grass of the savannah, but although they throw temper tantrums, their mothers resolutely refuse to tote them.

The refusal of mammalian animals to respond to the unnecessary demands of their offspring is probably universal. Parents thus avoid the intolerable burden of continued parenthood, and their offspring are encouraged to learn independence.

Good human parental care is no different from that given by other mammals, though the process may be spread out over 20 years. A baby who falls and hurts himself is immediately picked up and comforted by a fond and anxious mother. The baby grows into a small boy. For the fifth time in one afternoon, he comes howling to his mother because he has fallen in the garden. She tells him pretty firmly that he should not be so careless.

Setting Limits to Demands

A good parent offers loving and proper concern when it is

needed, and withholds it when it is not. A child makes constant demands to be looked after and for attention. Capable parents refuse their child's demands for unnecessary help. A parent is able to refuse help, and the child is able to accept such a refusal when love exists between them.

The state is more and more assuming the parental and helper role. Setting limits to demanding behavior becomes more difficult. The state's professional helpers—its schoolteachers, its social workers, its welfare officers and its doctors —do not easily establish affectionate bonds with a client or a patient that justifies the refusal to give help. It is often much more difficult to be firm with somebody else's recalcitrant child or somebody else's crotchety old mother than with one's near kin.

Professional helpers have difficulty in setting limits to the demands that are made upon them; they are sitting ducks for those who like to put others to work. Helpers often find themselves supplying help when they would rather not.

One young California drug addict literally ate a welfare worker. Although it is unusual for welfare workers to be made thus to supply lunch, it is certainly not unusual for welfare workers to be extremely misused.

It is said that in the days of slavery some men liked being slaves; and it is certainly true that many professional helpers enjoy self-sacrifice. But it is equally true that many of the more useful professional helpers do not. Mostly all professional helpers nowadays are government employees. Although some of them are quite prepared to incur unpopularity by saying no to the unnecessary demands made upon them, their employers are seldom so sanguine. Governments and government officials do not like unpopularity. They employ helpers to help, and they expect their helpers to do so.

Tryants, Rich and Poor

There is, of course, no limit to the futile help that helpers may be requested to give. In today's society, almost anyone can ask and receive. The rich have always been in a position to de-mand, as Ferdinand Lundberg points out in *The Rich and the Super Rich:*

> *The rich are especially enamored of medicine, and give heavily to their own hospitals and to medical research. Plainly, like the rest of us, they are seek-ing mundane salvation. But their faith in the powers of the doctors at times passeth all understanding. What I mean is illustrated by a story told me some years ago by an eminent internist, who complained that he had been detained for several hours on a sleeveless errand while many patients were in need of attention. He had been summoned with some ten or a dozen other specialists to attend a wealthy New York banker in his eighties who was very ill. It was obvious at a glance that the man was dying and yet members of the family walked about on tiptoe, with bated breath and looked upon the assembled doc-tors as a high priesthood capable of saving the wasted hulk—the patriarch and founder of the clan.*
>
> *The fees for this consultation, my annoyed in-formant told me, were bound to be astronomical, and the whole gathering obviously futile, an instance of medical fetishism. As E. M. Byers discovered, ex-pensive medical care cannot always save one.*

The rich have fallen into disfavor. We dislike, these days, the image of the rich Victorian housewife, tyrannizing the dozen underfed housemaids who catered to her whims. But not so very different is the present-day mother of six neglected children who colludes with her husband's drinking and man-ages never to pay the household bills. Such a woman not in-frequently has 15 or so different social agencies ministering to her and her family's needs. Usually, she is complaining, rude, and ungrateful toward her helpers.

Several studies have shown that about 5 percent of the

families in a community use up about half of that community's helping services. These studies noted that in spite of the large amount of help these multiproblem families were given, they persistently failed to respond to that help.

The cost of supplying help to help-demanding families is large. The cost alone in the salaries of social workers can be enormous. Over the many years that help is given to such families, dozens of professional helpers from various service agencies are involved. Two not atypical hard-core Toronto families received help, one for a period of 17 years and the other for a period of 23 years. The cost in the salaries of the social workers came to over $50,000 for each family—and the yearly salary of the social workers on which this estimate is based was around $1,700! Each of these families, therefore, had the equivalent of more than one full-time social worker looking after them during all the years the family received care.

Rx: More of the Same

If this kind of assistance did enable the more underprivileged members of society to manage their lives more competently, the money would be well spent. But there is scant evidence that this is so.

Why should the help be so unhelpful?

The efficacy of treatments is seldom questioned: if, for instance, pills are not working, then perhaps it is only because the dose needs to be doubled.

It is now accepted as a sociological truism that multiproblem families fail to be helped by the services they are rendered merely because they are not given enough of them. If social workers did not carry such large caseloads, it is claimed, they would then be able to counsel their clients more successfully and guide them toward self-sufficiency.

The New York State "Chemung County Study," designed to test the validity of this presumption, has been described by David Wallace, in the *Social Service Review*, as "one of the most rigorously designed evaluations of professional casework service yet attempted." Families receiving assistance were divided into two groups: (1) a demonstration group; and (2) a control group. The caseloads of the trained social-workers assigned to the demonstration group were kept light; moreover, these social workers received special cooperation from a wide range of community resources. The control group—the second group—received only the normal public assistance service.

Independent researchers measured the "family functioning" of the two groups before and after the two-year experiment. When the results were objectively evaluated, no significant changes were found in the family functioning of *either* group.

Not only is it difficult to demonstrate that conventional social work is useful, but it is difficult not to form the conclusion that the help of social agencies often serves only to confirm these struggling families in their dependent welfare way of life. The helpers are certainly kept busy, but the families do not change.

One of the most effective ways for multiproblem families to insure that their helpers stick relentlessly to their tasks is by having large numbers of uncared-for, unhappy, delinquent children. A recent study of multiproblem families in London, Ontario, showed that 45 percent of these families had five or more children, compared to 4 percent for the rest of the community. Only 21 percent of the fathers of these multiproblem families were in full-time employment; most of these families were entirely dependent upon the State for support. Because the children of these families learn helplessness rather than competence from their parents, the helplessness is likely to expand with each new generation.

Applying Parkinson's Law

Supply creates demand. Parkinson's famous law states that work expands to fill the time available. It is equally true that needs expand to match the help available. If more help is offered, more help will be used. It is difficult to know how useful this additional help will be.

Improvements in preventive medicine have successfully eliminated many infectious diseases. The lessening of these diseases has, needless to say, reduced the number of people with such diseases who require hospital admission. But the additional hospital beds thus made ·available have certainly not stayed empty.

SOURCES

Birt, Charles J.: "Family Centered Project." *Social Work*, 1 (4) 41 (1956).

Buell, Bradley, Beissner, Paul T., and Wedemyer, John W.: "Reorganizing to Prevent and Control Disordered Behavior." *Mental Hygiene*, **42** 155 (1958).

DeVore, Irven: Personal Communication, 1970.

Geismar, L. L., and Ayres, Beverley: *Families in Trouble*. St. Paul, Minn.: Family Centered Project, 1958.

Lundberg, Ferdinand: *The Rich and the Super Rich*. New York: Lyle Stuart, 1968.

Moore, A. M., and Robinson, W. J.: *Family Centered Project.* London (Ontario): United Community Services of Greater London, 1967.

Roseman, Renee: "Two Hardcore Families." (A manuscript thesis). School of Social Work, University of Toronto, 1960.

Schlesinger, Benjamin: *The Multiproblem Family: A Review and Annotated Bibliography*. Toronto: University of Toronto Press, 1970.

Toronto Daily Star: "Confessed Cannibal Hippie Charged in Montana Death." July 16, 1970.

Wallace, David: "The Chemung County Evaluation of Casework Service to Dependent Multiproblem Families." *Social Service Review*, **41** 379 (1967).

Warren, Roland L., and Smith, Jessie: "Casework Service to Chronically Dependent Multiproblem Families." *Social Service Review*, **37** 33 (1963).

Help Honking

Many of us like to promise help, but at someone else's expense. This is "help-honking." Politicians everywhere practice help honking the loudest. Here is a good example, as reported on the front page of the Toronto *Globe and Mail:*

SHULMAN SAYS MENTAL PATIENTS DENIED MEALS UNLESS
BEDS AND CLOTHES NEAT, TEETH CLEANED

Patients at the St. Thomas Psychiatric Hospital were being denied meals because they were not making their beds satisfactorily, not dressing neatly nor brushing their teeth, Dr. Morton Shulman charged yesterday.

The New Democratic Party member for High Park said that patients were forced to purchase their meals with tokens they earned for good behavior or work in the hospitals. Those who didn't earn enough tokens were denied meals, Dr. Shulman said.

He made an unannounced visit to the mental hospital yesterday morning after receiving a complaint about the Government-run institution's token system. At the end of his visit, hospital officials assured him that the token system for meals would be halted and that all patients will receive three meals a day, Dr. Shulman said.

The staffs of mental hospitals can be just as nasty as can other people. Patients in hospitals are particularly vulnerable to such nastiness, and it is right for the public to keep a watch-

184

ful eye open. But some complaints against staff are valid and some complaints are not.

For too long, mental hospitals have been making a great number of people helpless and dependent. Some of these hospitals are trying not to do this any longer; they are trying not to give unnecessary help. Few people would allow their teenage children to go around unwashed and smelling, or permit their children to leave their beds messed up for others to make. Yet this is the kind of behavior a hospital is asked to accept. This type of permissiveness is particularly unkind to patients, because when these patients get used to behaving like uncontrolled four-year-olds, nobody else wants to have anything to do with them.

Politically motivated help-honking only helps to establish the right of one group of society to exist at the expense of another, the right of patients to remain helpless and in need. Characteristic of the help-honking of politicians is their subsequent inability to provide adequate money for staff and facilities to cater to all those to whom these politicains have promised help.

While I was involved in running a rehabilitation unit in a large London mental hospital, I completely failed to persuade three sturdy patients to do anything toward helping in their own recovery. All three were quite content with their comfortable existence. It is difficult to discharge a man who has no job to go to. Social isolation, financial difficulties, and boredom will soon bring him back again to the hospital. Moreover, a man who has not worked for a long time seldom succeeds immediately in any full-time job. Pills will not make him get to work on time, nor will electroconvulsive therapy make him adjust to the unaccustomed activity of looking after himself. Only practice will.

Each of these three patients argued that he should not be asked to start work in the hospital, even for a few hours each week, since the hospital was only able to pay a few shillings in wages. In vain did I protest to each that the state already paid the considerable cost of his keep in hospital. Each maintained that this was only proper: he had a right to hospital care.

Not to be defeated, I wrote to the Department of Health and Social Security, and explained the predicament. I asked the department to withhold the weekly sickness payments to these three patients; and instead to allow us to use this money to pay these three patients for work done within the hospital. The department replied that since these patients were sick enough to be in a hospital, it was only right that they should continue to receive their sickness payments. This kind of "rightness" makes people stay sick.

The Code of Chronicity

Two American psychiatrists have compared the code that criminals use for thwarting police law enforcement to the code of behavior that mental hospital patients use to thwart the therapeutic activities of the staff. A new democratic regime introduced into a mental hospital has generally introduced more difficulties. These two American psychiatrists echo the sentiments of many hospital staffs when they write:

> *Patients have been well taught the principles of democracy, equality, therapeutic community, and the virtues of teamwork—so much so that they vociferously claim their inalienable right to behave as they choose but speak in whispers, if at all, about their corresponding obligations and duties.*
>
> *Hospital staffs have provided patients with numerous opportunities and forums to voice their gripes and participate in decisions affecting ward privileges and routine. However, under the banner of self-determination and therapeutic decision-making, patients are frequently granted privileges without corresponding obligations—a situation which has no comparable model in society. In society, a person gains the prerogative of being heard by assuming the*

*obligation of being productive and consistently ful-
filling the role of a responsible citizen. Where the
model breaks down in the mental hospital is precisely
at this point: patients are all too often granted representation without being expected to pay the taxes
of appropriate socialized, responsible behavior.*

It is in mental hospitals that the most disastrous effects of
treating people as helpless occur. The code of chronicity has
become widespread. It is not helpful to excuse people from
all responsibility. When the chronic sick can claim an in-
alienable right to be looked after, but can conveniently forget
an obligation to participate in their recovery, they stay disabled; and society is left with the rather tiresome burden of
having to support them.

The Paradox of Help

Help often proves unhelpful; and sometimes unhelpfulness
proves helpful. There are innumerable examples of this para-
dox. We pour aid and sympathy into some underdeveloped
countries; and they continue to be torn by internal strife and
to remain as socially chaotic and helpless as ever.

Against others, we gang up, and they unite and flourish.
Under the benign and helpful regime of a welfare state, the
suicide rate is high, and the attempted suicide rate far higher.
Under the most malignant and unhelpful of all regimes imag-
inable—the German concentration camps—suicide and attempted suicides were, in contrast, rare.

The terrible misfortunes of war have provided ample opportunities for the study of human beings under stressful conditions. L. B. Kalinowsky commented on these studies:

*Psychiatrists from many countries who studied this
question reported the astounding fact that there
seems to be hardly any limit to man's ability to
stand terrifying experiences.*

He suggests that "external pressures strengthen rather than weaken resistance against the expression of neurotic symptoms." When help is available, we break down more quickly.

In World War I, shell shock was accepted as an unavoidable reaction to explosions. Many soldiers invalided home from the front lines remained chronically shell-shocked. Toward the end of World War II, military psychiatrists had grown tougher. Soldiers with mental symptoms were treated near the front lines with the expectation that, after a short period of self-organization, they would return to duty. The satisfactory rehabilitation of psychiatric casualties rose immediately from 30 percent to 70 percent.

Most of us are much tougher than we think we are, or at least tougher than we are given credit for being by those who look after us. Government agencies predicted before World War II that if London were bombed, great numbers of people would flee from the city in panic, and that a tremendous outbreak of insanity would occur. Psychiatric casualties, it was anticipated, would outnumber physical casualties three to one. When the blitz did hit London, *there was no increase in the incidence of mental illness.* In fact, never have the hearts of Londoners so throbbed as one. Had the Germans dropped pound notes instead of bombs, the results might well have been more lethal. Too often injudicious helpfulness leaves in its wake a trail of disaster. We should be careful how we dish out help.

The extent to which helpers actually perpetuate the conditions for which they give help is a tricky sociological problem. Cripples make good beggars. In those countries where begging is common, it is by no means rare for parents to cripple their children so that they can beg more effectively. Most of us use our helplessness at some time as a means of getting other people to do things for us. The pretty girl whose car has a flat tire holds the jack upside down under the bumper until a man comes along and changes the tire.

Helpers who receive substantial rewards for their helpfulness have a vested interest in the continuance of helplessness. If it were possible to collect up all the nasty illnesses of mankind and put them back into Pandora's box, I and many thousands of others who are dependent upon sickness for our livelihood would, indeed, be worried. It is quite certain that the helping professions do create work for themselves.

Cushioning the Fall

Consider the teenage drug problem. Not only did the medical profession popularize the use of drugs in the first place, but doctors and other helpers do a lot—even if unwittingly—to encourage teenagers to use drugs.

A teenager stands at a crossroads in his life. He has reached an age when he would like to be independent, but he nevertheless remains reluctant to relinquish the support of his parents and of society on which he has always relied. To many such teenagers drugs appeal as the perfect solution. Because adults disapprove of drugs, by taking them the teenager can demonstrate his rebelliousness. At the same time, he makes himself ill—and thus manages to get himself looked after.

It is interesting to watch the teenagers at a pop festival waiting for the medical tent to be set up before they start shooting their drugs. They are making sure that someone will be there to rescue them—if they get lost on a psychedelic trip.

Especially on the American side of the Atlantic, large numbers of sociologists, psychologists, doctors, social workers, research workers, and administrators are employed on the problem of teenage drug addiction. If all the teenagers suddenly went straight, there would be catastrophic unemployment among such professional helpers. As long as these professional workers assiduously distribute pamphlets and hold innumerable conferences, lectures, and teach-ins, it is unlikely that the interest of the teenager in drugs will wane.

Or let us consider alcoholism. In terms of the havoc it causes, alcoholism is society's most serious mental health problem.

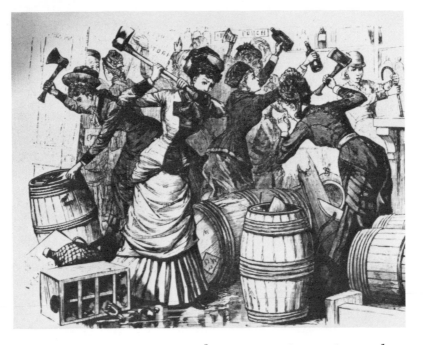

Temperance movements no longer campaign so vigorously to keep at least some of us on the water wagon.

Typically the alcoholic is a rather dependent man who marries a woman who is happy to mother him. The alcoholic likes being the bad little boy who needs looking after, and his wife likes her role of picking up the pieces after his drinking bouts. She is the gallant mainstay of the family. The more robust woman quickly rebels when her husband gets drunk, but the alcoholic's wife, though she belittles him for his drinking, continues to condone it. She condones it, that is, until his wits become so befuddled with alcohol that he loses his job, he gets dirty and smells, he has temper tantrums and beats her up. The rescuing game is then no longer worth the candle and she quits.

The helping professionals now take over. They label the alcoholic as sick, which excuses him from responsibility for his behavior. Like the alcoholic's wife, the helping professionals continue to rescue the alcoholic from the consequences of his drinking. Repeatedly, after his last few dollars have turned into cheap wine, they fix him up with a bed, more food, and more money. The alcoholic can remain inebriated, unencumbered by the necessity of fending for himself.

Of course professional helpers, like the alcoholic's wife, have a limit to their patience. In the end the detoxification center, the hospital emergency department, and the hostel all ignominiously throw him out. But every city in North America has so many helping agencies that the alcoholic can continue to provide himself with help until he dies of drink, or until he becomes so mentally and physically incapacitated that he requires permanent institutional care.

Perhaps there would be fewer alcoholics if there were fewer alcoholics' wives. Would there also be fewer alcoholics if there were fewer professional helpers? This is an impossible question to answer, but it is possible to hazard a guess.

Epidemiologists keep track of the number of alcoholics in the community. They derive their figures, at least in part, from the number of people dying each year from cirrhosis of the liver and not from the number of alcoholics receiving treatment. Taking this into consideration would most certainly boost their figures upward.

There has, in all Western Countries over the last few decades, been a rise in the prevalence of alcoholism. There are at least two good reasons for this increase. One, our growing affluence means that we all have more money to spend on alcohol, and two, the brass band temperance movements now no longer campaign so vigorously to keep at least some of us on the water wagon. But it is my guess that professional helpers—with their relentless propensity to infantilize the alcoholic and keep him helpless and dependent—have at least in part contributed to our increasing rates of alcoholism. In Sweden, where professional helpers are the most available, the incidence of alcoholism has risen 424 percent in the last decade.

Help: A Bottomless Well?

Very large numbers of people are involved in supplying health. In the United States, 3 million people now work in the health industry, and this industry has a vested interest in keeping sickness going. Moreover, professional helpers have their own emotional needs to be helpful, and being helpful often turns out to be very different from being useful or constructive.

Everybody expects helpers to be helpful, including, of course, helping themselves. So willy-nilly, a helper is forced into making placating gestures. He makes it appear as if he is trying to prevent suicide by locking up his depressed patients. He prescribes pills to patients which often end up doing more harm than good. He refers a patient with insoluble problems to some other helpers, and so dispatches his patient on a pointless merry-go-round of appointments. Never, never, never does a helper just confess that he cannot help in any way.

Providing useful help is often hard work both for the helper and the person to be helped. Hard work does not come all that naturally to many of us.

Many of us do not want to be bothered with the self-discipline that health requires, nor with the tiresome effort that may be needed for the recovery from illness. We prefer to rely on magic pills, and to enjoy just being looked after. Prescribing pills is easy for the doctor, and although looking after people may be dull, it is considerably less hard work for the helper than the creative effort needed either to encourage people to get better, or even to urge the patient to opt out of what has become an unfruitful situation. Helpers and the recipients of help are often only too happy to settle for the easy way.

Missing the Trees for the Forest

The sick and helpless wait in increasing numbers for professional helpers to get them better. And the helpers, often not really knowing how to help, get sick with identity crises. Or they manage to sidestep the difficult problem of helping by championing dubious treatments, writing books, performing esoteric research, attending far-away conventions, or holding endless meetings with their therapeutic teams. While the helpless wait to be helped, the helpers are busy doing something else.

Meanwhile, those who are old and feeble or who are by sickness truly handicapped, often end up by getting very little of the useful help they really need.

SOURCES

Crook, Farrell: "Mental Patients Denied Meals: Shulman Assails Use of Tokens." *Globe and Mail* (Toronto), June 17, 1970.

Gil, David G.: *Violence Against Children.* Cambridge: Harvard University Press, 1970.

Kalinowsky, L. B.: "Problems of War Neurosis in the Light of Experience in Other Countries." *American Journal of Psychiatry,* **107** 340 (1950).

Lohman, Hans: *Mental Health and Human Environment.* Report No. 30, National Board of Health and Welfare. Stockholm: 1972.

Ludwig, Arnold M., and Farrelly, Frank: "The Code of Chronicity." *Archives of General Psychiatry,* **15** 562 (1966).

Miller, Miles D.: "The Mobile Psychiatric Team: Peacetime Uses of Combat Psychiatry." *American Journal of Psychiatry,* **121** Supplement May 1965.

Wolfenstein, Martha: *Disaster: A Psychological Essay.* London: Routledge and Kegan Paul, 1957.

Dabbling with Death

Many of us like being looked after, and all of us like having our own way: "If you leave me," threatens the patient, "I'll kill myself." Threatening suicide has always been a popular method of getting one's own way. It has now become an effective method of getting oneself looked after.

Suicide is common. It is the tenth most common cause of death in Western countries. At one time not too long ago, suicide was not considered to be a medical problem. But because mentally sick people have a slightly higher suicide rate than others, suicide has become the particular concern of the psychiatrist.

Can Suicide Be Prevented?

Psychiatrists and society in general usually regard the prevention of suicide as the job of the psychiatrist. There is little evidence he can do so. People kill themselves for many and varied reasons; and perhaps most of these reasons are beyond the competence of the psychiatrist.

Analysis of the suicide rates for England and the United States for this century develops three very noticeable facts:

1. There is a close connection between a rapid increase in unemployment and a high suicide rate.

2. During the years of the two major world wars— 1914–1918 and 1940–1945—suicide rates fell.

3. Neither the introduction of shock treatment in the

*1930s nor the introduction of the anti-depressants
in the middle 1950s appears to have had any noticeable effect on the rate of mental health cure.*

Psychiatrists cannot prevent economic recessions. On the contrary, to the extent that costly psychiatric services drain government resources from use in areas which are more economically productive, such costly psychiatric services merely compound economic ills. Non-productive government spending helps increase inflation, which, in turn, leads to economic recession, fewer jobs, and more suicides.

Wars seem to keep people happier; at least, fewer people kill themselves during wars. In all the countries involved in World War II, suicide rates dropped as much as 20 to 50 percent during the war's duration.

The introduction of penicillin caused a remarkable drop in deaths due to many bacterial diseases. But the introduction of drug treatments for depression has not caused a noticeable decline in deaths by suicide. It seems reasonable to conclude that psychiatric treatments are not very effective in preventing suicide.

Northern Ireland has a National Health Service, with plenty of doctors to give shock treatment or to prescribe anti-depressants. Yet its suicide rate has climbed for the past 25 years—until the outbreak of violence between the Catholics and the Protestants in the summer of 1969. Then the suicide rate fell dramatically. The reduction in suicides and in reported cases of depression has been especially striking in the areas where most of the violence has occurred. A good fight seems to cheer many people better than do the pills or the ministrations of psychiatrists.

Psychiatrists have not even been successful in preventing their hospitalized patients from killing themselves. It is difficult for the psychiatrist to know which, if any, of his patients will kill themselves. Except, perhaps, for severe depression, no particular mental disorder is associated with a particularly high risk of suicide. Disconcertingly, many mentally sick peo-

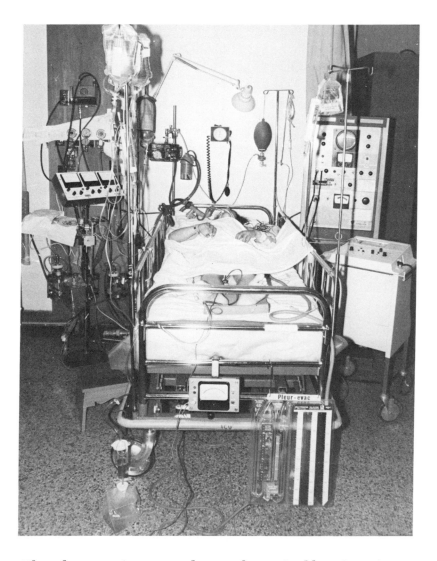

*Though many of us now take overdoses of tablets, few of us
expect to die from them. We rely on the hospital to save us.
This woman has taken an overdose, and much skilled time and
expensive equipment is required to save her life.*

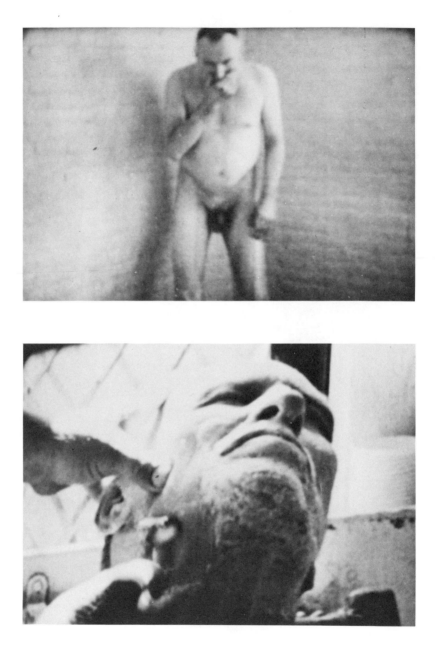

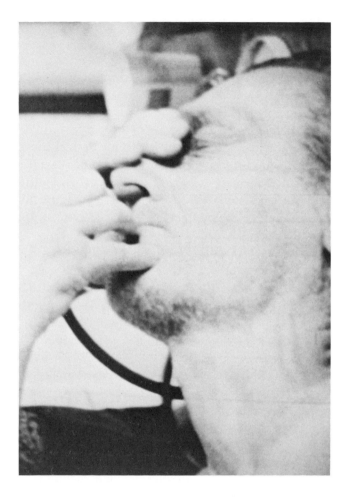

This man was a patient of the Bridgewater Mental Hospital, Massachusetts, in 1967. He was kept naked in his room so that he would not use his clothes to strangle himself. He was shaved by an intern, since he was not permitted to handle his own razor. And he was force-fed through a tube, for otherwise he would have starved himself to death. When hospitals stop using these unpleasant suicide precautions, the suicide rate of their patients goes down.

ple kill themselves at a time when they appear to be recovering rather than when they appear most ill.

Protecting the Sick from Themselves

To play safe, for years mental hospitals kept their patients in locked wards to guard against suicide. Knives and forks, razors, belts, ties, and all other potentially dangerous objects— sometimes even clothes—were prohibited to these patients. Persons considered to be particularly dangerous to themselves were made to sit all day on special benches where they could be guarded by the hospital attendants. These patients were even accompanied to the toilet. In spite of these stringent precautions, patients still found ingenious ways of cheating their guards and caretakers and of doing themselves in.

So farcical had all these precautions become that it was a great relief when a few brave psychiatrists opened their wards and stopped bothering about protecting their patients at all. For years, the suicide rate in English mental hospitals had remained steady at about 50 per 100,000 patients per year. In 1953, after many English hospitals had opened their wards and curtailed strict surveillance, the suicide rate dropped to 27.3 per 100,000 patients. Although the rate has crept up again to 38 suicides per 100,000, this rate is still lower than that when hospitals were concentrating upon not letting their patients kill themselves. The figures for American mental hospitals have followed much the same pattern.

It is hardly surprising that when the unhappy were no longer locked up in drab wards for their own protection, with their cordless pajamas slipping down around their ankles all day, they felt a bit better and less like killing themselves. Interestingly, the introduction of electroconvulsive therapy, the psychiatrist's favorite treatment for depression, didn't make a scrap of difference in the suicide rate among patients in mental hospitals.

Fear of Malpractice Suits

We live in a blame-shifting society. We prefer when possible to assign blame and responsibility to professional helpers and institutions. Although it is fairly obvious that psychiatrists and hospitals cannot prevent a patient who is determined to kill himself from doing so, doctors and hospitals are often held responsible for these deaths. Indeed, in attempting to thwart such suicides, doctors have often quite unwarrantedly interfered with individual freedom. In the United States, one in three hospital suicides is followed by a malpractice suit against either the hospital or the doctor.

In November, 1970, a 21-year-old man was awarded nearly $48,000 in damages after he jumped off the roof of a London hospital and broke his neck. He had been admitted to the hospital after having taken an overdose of pills. He managed to leave a busy 27-bed ward unnoticed by climbing through a window. The judge said that the accident would not have happened had the three nurses on duty kept their patient under closer observation. The nurses who were held responsible for this patient's self-inflicted injury could not, even after a lifetime of constructive hard work, save as much money as this man earned by his one destructive act.

Forty-eight thousand dollars is a lot of money; but on the American side of the Atlantic such an escapade might well win a patient a half million dollars or so. The next time you are in a hospital and the nurses refuse to let you look out of the window, remember that it is not only your neck that they are worried about.

Many psychiatrists are easily made anxious—if not intimidated—by the critical remarks of coroners or by threatened litigation by relatives. They do not feel secure unless their patients are safely locked up and guarded by a diligent nursing staff. Then, in case of a successful suicide, they can claim that they did everything humanly possible to prevent it. This is crazy.

Who Protects the Protectors?

Not only does locking up patients for their own protection actually increase the chances that they *will* kill themselves, but these are not the people in our society who are the most likely to commit suicide. The suicide rate for doctors is high; for psychiatrists, it is particularly so.

In fact, in the United States, psychiatrists commit suicide at nearly twice the rate of patients in mental hospitals.

If we really think it is necessary to protect people against themselves, and that locking people up keeps them safe, then it must be regarded as irresponsible not to incarcerate psychiatrists in their own mental hospitals. I would not like this very much myself.

There is only one sure way to prevent a man from killing himself: he must be helped to find his life more meaningful. This is much easier said than done. Certainly, it does not add meaning to a man's life to confine him in a locked ward, to survey him as he sits on the toilet, to take away his clothes, to count his cutlery after every meal, and to subject him to all the other jiggery-pokeries still used in many hospitals as a precaution against suicide.

Only when society stops holding hospitals and psychiatrists responsible for the suicides of their patients will these silly precautions finally stop. Even psychiatrists—provided they are not held responsible for other people's actions over which they have no control—may cheer up a little, and stop killing themselves so often.

The Suicide Threat

Threatening suicide is common behavior; but threatening suicide is very much different from committing it. The threat is a convenient and effective way of making others do what you want them to.

"If you don't help me, I'll have to end it all"; or "If you don't give me what I want, I'll kill myself." Such threats are most commonly made to families, to those with whom such emotional appeals are expected to be effective. Suicide threats are also public demands for attention or sympathy—for instance, the dramatic threat to jump off a high building, staged before a gasping crowd.

Sometimes such threats are unsuccessful. A disablement case had been appealed, and was tried before Lord Justice Edmund Davies. As the honorable justice pronounced a judgment unfavorable to the plaintiff, the man jumped up, dramatically poured several tablets from a bottle, and swallowed them. The judge paused momentarily, while the man ran from the room shouting, "I might as well end it all now."

A few minutes later, the plaintiff was returned to the court room. He ostentatiously swallowed more pills. Unperturbed, the judge asked calmly if the plaintiff had anything to say. The man replied: "It does not matter, I shall be dead before you can write out the judgment."

He was not. Whatever the pills were, they were harmless. But few people either in public life or in private would retain his composure as did Lord Davies in the face of such a threat.

Swallowing overdoses of medication is the commonest way of making blackmailing suicide gestures. At the end of the 1940s, doctors were prescribing barbiturates for anxiety and insomnia—and their patients were taking overdoses of them. For instance, the number of patients admitted to the Edinburgh Royal Infirmary for barbiturate overdose rose from 10 in 1945 to 350 in 1960.

Many more drugs for the mind are now available, and the number of attempted suicides has continued to increase. By 1966, 10 percent of all admissions to English hospitals were for self-poisoning. By 1970, in some parts of Britain, half the admissions to medical wards of women between the ages of 15 and 40 were for an overdose of pills. I have not been able to find reliable figures for the incidence of self-poisoning in the United States, but it is quite certain that more people than ever are now taking overdoses of drugs.

Emergency Relief

A fundamental tenent of good medicine is that prevention is better than cure. In discussing what to do about would-be suicides, Professor Kessel takes the traditional view that more help is needed:

> *It is, however, essential to provide the patient with an alternative way of securing support at the very moment when he feels he must have it. Emergency services must be offered to provide emergency relief. The patient must know that he can get help without having to pay the price of self-poisoning or self-injury.*

Such emergency services would indeed be useful if the need for help was always finite. A distressed man could attend an emergency clinic, receive the necessary help, and then leave without having to poison himself. But often the need for help is infinite. The more help one is given, the more helpless he becomes, and the more help he then needs.

An English psychiatrist tested Professor Kessel's hypothesis that the availability of emergency relief would reduce the incidence of self-poisoning. With the aid of a grant from the Nuffield Foundation, this doctor provided an emergency call service making several social workers available 24 hours a day for 97 patients who had taken overdoses. Each patient was eligible to utilize this service for six months following his overdose. An equal number of similar patients received no such service. At the end of the study, the professional workers were exhausted, but the number of patients in the two groups who had taken additional overdoses was about the same. In the control group, 19 had taken one or more overdoses; in the serviced group, 17 had taken one or more overdoses. Providing emergency services to prevent attempted suicide is probably not a profitable use of professionals' time.

But arguments still continue as to the usefulness of suicide prevention programs. Unlike most other countries, England has been lowering its suicide rate since the middle of the 1960s, without either a war or an economic boom to help. In 1953, "The Samaritans" was founded in England to provide support for people who thought about killing themselves. Today, the Samaritans provide an extensive telephone support service for would-be suicides. Samaritans and doctors alike claim credit for the fall in England's suicide rate.

Putting one's head in the gas oven was for many years the commonest way by which the English chose to commit suicide. Following in the wake of the widespread prescription by doctors of barbiturates and other "drugs for the mind," poisoning with these drugs gained ascendancy as the number one method. In the last decade, suicide by such poisoning continued to rise, while the number of suicide deaths by coal-gas poisoning took a deep plunge. It is this fall in the number of deaths by coal-gas poisoning which accounts for the recent fall in England's suicide rate.

Curious about the drop in gas-inhalation deaths, I asked the British Gas Board what they thought might be the reason. They explained that, during the last decade, the amount of lethal carbon monoxide in gas had been gradually reduced. In many areas, it was no longer possible to kill oneself by turning on the gas, and then putting one's head in the oven and breathing deeply. It is, then, the Gas Council, not Britain's suicide prevention programs, which must be credited with the drop in English suicides.

The suicidal gesture that most often accompanies suicidal threats is the taking of an overdose of pills. Seldom are such gestures meant to be fatal; yet sometimes by accident, they are. While it may be safe to take 100 times the normal dosage of one sort of pill, much smaller numbers of another may be fatal. Undoubtedly, the sub-lethal dose is sometimes miscalculated.

Suicide threats are a popular and effective way of exploiting the benefits of the welfare state. The alcoholic, without funds for a night's lodging, uses the threat as a ploy to

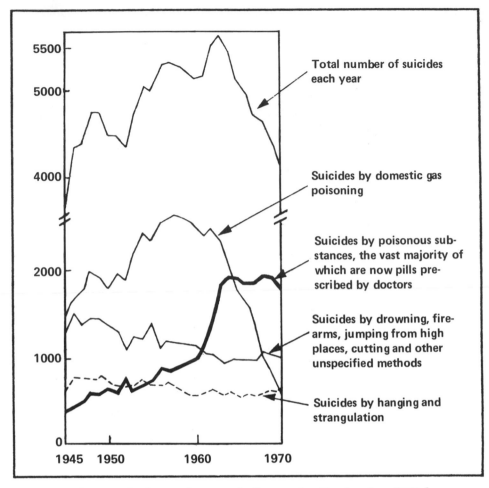

5500 —
5000 —
4000 —
2000 —
1000 —
0 —

1945 1950 1960 1970

Total number of suicides each year

Suicides by domestic gas poisoning

Suicides by poisonous substances, the vast majority of which are now pills prescribed by doctors

Suicides by drowning, firearms, jumping from high places, cutting and other unspecified methods

Suicides by hanging and strangulation

This graph shows the suicide figures for England and Wales between 1950 and 1970. The sharp drop in deaths due to gas inhalation between 1960 and 1970 must be credited to the Gas Council, which during this time had been gradually reducing the amount of lethal carbon monoxide in the gas.

get into a hospital. The amphetamine addict threatens his doctor with suicide if he does not get a renewal of his supplies.

Few doctors whose patients blackmail them with threats of suicide are prepared to exercise the imperturbability of

Lord Davies. A suicide threat is generally accepted as indicative of mental illness; the failure of a doctor to respond to such a threat is construed as professional negligence. From the doctor's point of view, it is better to capitulate rather than be sued by surviving relatives. Moreover, a doctor has been trained to respond.

The Plea for Baby Help

Psychiatry teaches that suicide threats are cries for help, and so they are. But seldom are they cries for *constructive* help. Constructive help—if it can be obtained at all—can usually be had without the aid of such behavior. A suicide threat is a demand for Baby Help; and the helper is made to help in a manner which he himself does not consider useful.

If, as Professor Kessel and others have suggested, emergency services are established for the purpose of lessening the incidence of self-poisoning, then it seems inevitable that those providing these services will be blackmailed, even more than they are at present, into giving help against their better judgment. "I'll kill myself" will become a yet more effective method of getting one's own way. The establishment of such services is likely to increase—not decrease—the incidence of suicidal threats and gestures.

The United States has a tradition of violence going back to its frontier days. The tradition carries over into the methods used by suicides. In England, before the Gas Council started to reduce the carbon monoxide in household gas, quiet deaths by gas poisoning accounted for 40 percent of all suicides, and death from gun-shot wounds for only 3 percent. In contrast, fewer than 1 percent of American suicides use gas; nearly half shoot themselves.

Americans can buy guns more easily than schoolboys in certain countries can buy cap pistols. If the people of the United States really want to reduce its suicide rate, it will more likely succeed in doing so by passing strict laws of gun control than by providing ever more expensive psychiatric services for suicide prevention.

SOURCES

Bewley, Thomas: "Estimate of Incidence of Drug Abuse in the United Kingdom." *Bulletin of Narcotics,* **13** (1967).

Blachly, P. M., Disher, William, and Roduner, G.: "Suicide by Physicians." *Bulletin of Suicidology* (National Institute of Mental Health), Dec. 1968.

British Medical Journal: "Suicide Among Doctors." **1** 789 (1964).

Bureau of Labor Statistics, U.S. Department of Labor: *Employment and Earnings.* **18** (8), Feb. 1972.

Bureau of the Census: *Historical Statistics of the United States, Colonial Times to 1957.* Washington, D.C.: Government Printing Office, 1960.

Copstick, Alan: "Recognition of Emotional Disturbance and the Prevention of Suicide." *British Medical Journal,* **1** 1179 (1960).

Davidson, Henry A.: "Suicide in Hospital." *Hospitals: Journal of the American Hospital Association,* **43** (22) 55 (1969).

Department of Employment and Productivity: *British Labour Statistics: Historical Abstract, 1886–1968.* London: Her Majesty's Stationery Office, 1971.

————: *Annual Reports* (1968–1971), London: Her Majesty's Stationery Office.

DeSole, Daniel E., Singer, Philip, and Aronson, Samuel: "Suicide and Role Strain Among Physicians." *International Journal of Social Psychiatry,* **15** 294 (1969).

Hicks, Robert C., and Chowdhury, Nilima: "Evaluation of an After Care Service for Patients Repeatedly Attempting Suicide." In press.

Kessel, Neil: "The Respectability of Self-Poisoning and the Fashion for Survival." *Journal of Psychosomatic Research,* **10** 29 (1966).

————: "Self-Poisoning." *British Medical Journal,* **4** 1268 (1965).

———— and Grossman, G.: "Suicide in Alcoholics." *British Medical Journal* **2** 1671 (1961).

———— and McCullock, W.: "Repeated Acts of Self-Poisoning and Self-Injury." *Proceedings of the Royal Society of Medicine,* **59** 89 (1966).

Lancet: "Help for the Despairing. The Work of the Samaritans." 2 1102 (1962).

Litman, R.: Quoted by Henry A. Davidson in "Suicide in Hospital." *Hospitals: Journal of the American Hospital Association,* **43** (22) 55 (1969).

Lyons, H. A.: "Depressive Illness and Oppression in Belfast." *British Medical Journal,* 1 342 (1972).

Matthew, H.: "Poisoning in the Home by Medicaments." *British Medical Journal,* 2 788 (1966).

Medical Protection Society (Great Britain): *Annual Report for 1970.*

Mills, Ivor M.: "Human Lemmings Escape from the Reality of Life." *The Times* (London), May 30, 1970.

Mitchell, B. R.: *Abstract of British Historical Statistics.* London: Cambridge University Press, 1962.

O'Driscoll, James.: "£19,000 for Suicide Risk Patient." *Daily Telegraph* (London), Nov. 26, 1970.

Perr, Irwin N.: "Liability of Hospital and Psychiatrist in Suicide." *American Journal of Psychiatry,* **122** 631 (1965).

Registrar General: *Annual Reports: Northern Ireland.* Belfast: Her Majesty's Stationery Office, 1945–1971.

————: *Statistical Reviews of England and Wales* (for the years 1945, 1960, 1967, 1970). London: Her Majesty's Stationery Office.

Ross, Mathew: "Suicide Among College Students." *American Journal of Psychiatry,* **126** 220 (1969).

Slater, Eliot, and Roth, Martin: Mayer-Gross Clinical Psychiatry. London: Bailliere, Tindall and Cassell, 1961.

Stengel, Erwin: *Suicide and Attempted Suicide.* London: Penguin Books, 1964.

Temby, W. D.: "Suicide." In *Problems of the Student.* Ed. G. B. Blain and C. C. McArthur. New York: Appleton-Century-Crofts, 1961.

U. S. Department of Health, Education and Welfare, National Centers for Health Statistics: *Suicide in the United States, 1950–1960. Series 20. No. 5.*

————: *Annual Summary in the United States, 1970. Vital Statistics Report 19* (13). Sept. 1971.

World Health Organization: "Mortality for Suicide." *Epidemiological and Vital Statistics.* Report. 9 243 (1956).

Yessler, Paul G., Gibbs, James J., and Becker, Herman A.: "On the Communication of Suicidal Ideas." *Archives of General Psychiatry,* 3 612 (1960).

Delivering Health

All professions are a conspiracy against the laity.

GEORGE BERNARD SHAW

Government departments of health are perhaps jealous of the budgets, even larger than their own, which are awarded to the departments of defense. At least they make the health care they provide for us sound like ballistic missiles, and our health care now comes to us by health-care delivery systems. The next three chapters are about these systems, the deliverers and their targets.

Traditionally, health was a private concern between a man and his physician. If a sick man had money, he employed a physician to help him to recover. If he had no money, then the physician—if he was generous—looked after him for nothing. By the 19th century, this system was breaking down; the poor in many of the big cities of Europe were far too numerous to be cared for by personal charity. In 1849, Bismarck stated:

The social insecurity of the workers is the real cause of their being an insecurity to the state.

Because most every government wanted its working class to be healthy, the government had to do something about providing medical care.

In the late 1880s, after 40 years of struggle, Bismarck,

who was an arch-conservative and a detester of socialism, expertly manipulated the Reichstag into establishing the first compulsory nationwide insurance scheme for the working classes. The poor in Germany were protected against accidents, sickness, and old age. Bismarck's paternalistic socialism served as a model for other European countries, and also serves as an uncomfortable source of anxiety for the American Medical Association.

Lessening the Financial Burden

All Western countries have now developed an assortment of schemes to provide medical care for those who need it but who cannot afford to pay for it, and these schemes have partly succeeded in providing such care. They have lessened people's fear of financial ruin through illness, and they have warmed the cold hand of charity upon which many of the poor have had to rely for medical care.

Nevertheless, most of the optimism with which these schemes were introduced has proved unwarranted. The Beveridge Report, which fathered the British National Health Service, found that the health of Britain was poor. The report assumed that the cost of the health service would decline as soon as the backlog of needy cases was taken care of. The cost of the British National Health Service rose nearly 1,000 percent in its first 20 years, which shows how unsupported was this optimism.

Most schemes for health care have left their authors disappointed, the recipients of the care disgruntled, and their sponsoring government in a state of financial embarrassment.

Present health care hinges around the relationship between a doctor and his patients. Because I am a doctor, I will choose the important consideration of pay arrangements as a means of classifying the various ways of delivering health. There is no satisfactory way in which a doctor can be paid for the services he renders to a patient, though certainly some ways of paying him turn out to be more disastrous than others. The four common ways in which doctors get paid are by:

(1) private fee (with or without insurance cover)
(2) capitation fee
(3) fee for service
(4) salary

There are pros and cons in all these methods of payment.

The Private Fee System

Payment by private fee is the traditional way by which a patient pays his doctor. It has the advantage that the doctor and patient fall easily into a contractual relationship with each other. The patient pays the doctor to help him to recover. The extent of the service that the patient expects to receive, and the time and energy that the doctor expects to devote to the patient, are defined by the size of the fee. If the patient places enormous demands on the doctor, the doctor increases his fee. Because he pays for his own treatment, the patient invests more interest in his recovery. He gets better more quickly.

Doctors are thus encouraged to provide the services that their patients want. Mrs. Green may sell the best lettuce; Mr. Brown, the best potatoes. One doctor may be good with broken hearts; another, with anal warts. By practicing the kind of medicine he is best at, a doctor, under the fee system, entices patients to consult him. And these patients are pleased to use that doctor's skills.

But private payment of the doctor has big disadvantages. Medical treatment is becoming more complicated and more expensive. Many people, especially at a time when they are ill, cannot afford to pay for treatment. And undoubtedly, private medicine encourages doctors to foster *unnecessary* treatments. "Health" can be made to yield vast profits.

The Pursuit of Health

The health industry extols its achievements. Nowadays, many of us expect to be healthy all the time. The World Health

Organization sets the tone by defining health as a "state of complete physical, social and emotional well-being," a real pie-in-the-sky definition.

More realistically, health has been described as a hypo-chrondriacal delusion. Few of us are prepared to take the time and trouble to obtain the rude physical health of an Olympic athlete; and even athletes catch colds. Life is a terrifying event. Our fellow human beings are often unpredictable, ruthless, downright bad. They create situations that are far from conducive to complete emotional well-being. At best, we can make only a precarious adjustment to life. Often, we both feel vulnerable and are vulnerable. We also feel deprived, frightened, uncertain.

Few of us sustain perfect health for very long—95 percent of people interviewed in two London boroughs reported some health complaint within the previous two weeks. Other surveys have shown that only about a third of recognizable illnesses are actually seen by a doctor. Mostly, people just wait for their illnesses to get better.

Treatment for Treatment's Sake

Doctors, depending for their livelihood upon their patients being sick, have discouraged such hopeful passivity. Doctors in the past have certainly encouraged both illness and treatment; and many doctors, especially where much of medical practice remains private, still do. We have seen how the normal physiological irregularities of the bowel were labeled constipation, and required vigorous treatment; and we have also seen how normally large tonsils were—and still are—held to be diseases, and are declared candidates for removal.

There are a host of minor illnesses from which we can recover perfectly well on our own but which now have been made to require the attention of a doctor. Today, we are taught that our emotional problems also require a doctor's aid. So effective has medical propaganda been that patients have come to believe that treatments are imperative. Only through treatment can life, limb, and happiness be preserved.

Once it was just illnesses like colds which "properly treated" provided a large chunk of the family doctor's income. But the days of such cottage industry have been left far behind; the health business is now big business. As in most other things, the United States leads the way. Health is the third largest industry in the U.S., with only agriculture and construction ahead of it. And health is quickly catching up with them, too. In 1940, Americans spent about $4 billion, or nearly 4 percent of their gross national product, on their health; in 1965, $38.9 billion, or 5.9 percent of the GNP; and in 1969, $67.8 billion, or 7 percent. The cost of America's health is going up fast.

Just as the car industry used built-in obsolescence and the continual production of new models to insure a booming continuation of its business, so does the health industry continually devise new and more costly treatments. It encourages in its consumers both doctor and treatment dependency.

A Word for Therapeutic Restraint

Sickness has great sentimental appeal. It is difficult for anybody to resist the blandishments of the health industry. And death is the bogey of our society. We find it difficult to let someone die even when he wants to. One chest surgeon, appalled by the expensive and often painful techniques that his colleagues were using to prolong the lives of the dispirited elderly, declared that he will have "Do Not Open" tattooed on his chest.

Few doctors are prepared to encourage such therapeutic restraint. Medical science is developing techniques to keep a person or the bits of a person alive for almost an indefinite period. Cryogenic interment now aims to help the rich escape the call of death altogether. For a package deal of $50,000 a dying body is frozen in liquid nitrogen. When cures are discovered for the fatal disease, the body will be unfrozen and treated. It is unlikely that such individuals will ever need

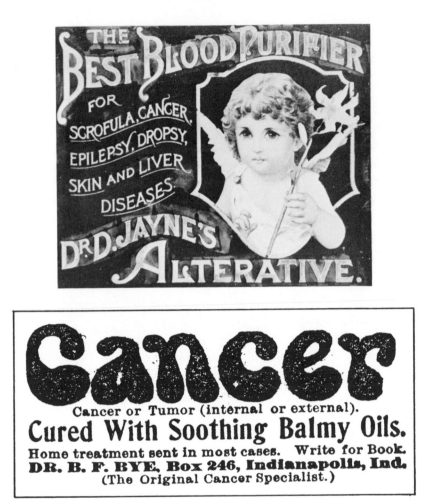
Old magazines are full of doctor's advertisements which make claim to all kinds of incredible cures. Though doctors are no longer allowed to advertise their cures to the public, many still practice their "favorite treatments."

the $10,000 that the Cryogenic Society recommends be put in trust for the frigidly interred against the day he is resurrected from the cryostat.

But other techniques are proving more successful. After a man has creamed his brain in a traffic accident, respirators, tube feeding, and devoted nursing can keep his insensate body alive for years. He will never recover consciousness. But nobody will turn off the switch of the respirator that supplies his body with life. Brilliant, though perhaps somewhat macabre, surgical techniques now make it possible to replace some of our damaged giblets with new ones.

Health Insurance

Such treatments—indeed all forms of modern medical attention—are cripplingly expensive. When medicine is private, most middle-class people try to protect themselves with a health insurance policy from the misfortune of having to pay medical bills. Blue Cross is the largest and best known of the companies that supply such policies. These private insurance companies pay on the basis of "reasonable charges" presented by the doctor. The doctor, knowing that some faceless insurance company will pay his bill, regards as "reasonable" whatever sum he can get away with.

Just as a garage charges more for repairs when an insurance company is paying the bill, so does a doctor. And just as a car owner often demands a perfect job on crumpled fenders when the repairs are covered by insurance—but is quite content to live with the dents when they are not—so does a patient often demand much more detailed medical attention once his health care is insured. These increased patient demands, combined with payment of "reasonable charges," soon raises the cost of health care. Inevitably, this raises the cost of health insurance premiums.

In 1960, an average American father with two children paid $408 in health insurance premiums and medical bills. In 1969, he paid $676. The size of that increase was three times that of the cost-of-living increase during the same period. Health insurance premiums are now very expensive, and Blue Cross has now become a heavy cross to bear.

Because of the ever increasing cost of health care, the old and the poor are unable to pay their health bills. In 1966, the Federal Government, faced with a breakdown in medical care for the aging, introduced Medicare. The states, in turn, supplied Medicaid. Medicare helps finance the medical care of those over 65 years of age; Medicaid provides medical aid to the indigent. The American Medical Association, always suspicious of even any hint of socialized medicine, at first viewed these two schemes with discomfort. Its fears were unnecessary.

Medicare and Medicaid

Like the private insurance companies, Medicare and Medicaid pay on the basis of reasonable charges submitted by the doctor. The doctors again edged up their fees so that both Medicare and Medicaid turned out to be a bonanza for the health industry. The *British Medical Journal,* perhaps rather smugly, was soon referring to them as "America's unhealthy twins."

The annual cost of Medicare has climbed from 1.3 billion dollars in 1967, to 3.2 billion in 1968, and to 5.5 billion in 1969. In 1970, the cost rose to 8 billion dollars. Medicaid is costing twice as much as expected. In 1969, 8,000 American doctors earned at least $25,000 each in fees from these two schemes. Two doctors received $375,000 each for treating patients in a nursing home which they themselves owned.

Private medicine, especially when covered by insurance, soon makes medical care so expensive that it cripples those individuals or governments who have to pay for it. In the United States, more than a third of the cost of medical care is now borne by government; but care has become so expensive that the country cannot afford to provide anything like proper medical care for its needy. Nor can middle-class Americans afford to buy proper care for themselves. In July 1969, President Nixon described the situation as a massive crisis in health care. There is no reason to expect that the system of private medicine will produce anything but an ever worsening crisis.

Spending money on expensive treatment is, of course, not a good way to provide any nation with good health care. Judged by mortality figures, United States citizens do not appear to be particularly healthy. American have an average life expectancy several years shorter than the citizens of most European countries. Infant mortality in the United States is 21 per 1,000 compared to 18 per 1,000 in England, and 13 per 1,000 in Norway. Maternal mortality in the U.S. is twice that of Sweden.

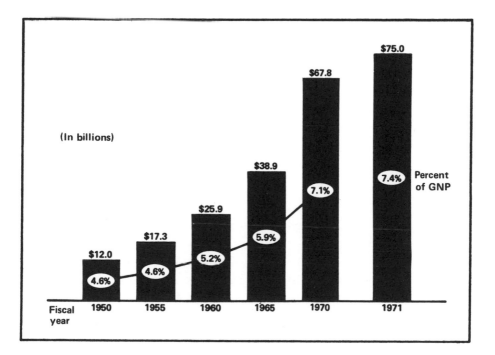

This chart shows U.S. health expenditures (private and public), and their percentages of the gross national product for selected fiscal years between 1950 and 1971. The cost of health care continues to rise.

Yet the United States spends far more on health per capita than does any other country. If the British were to spend as much per head on health as do Americans, British taxes would have to go up still another 10 percent. Both Poland and Czechoslovakia have a lower mortality rate than Britain, yet they spend even a smaller percentage of their gross national product on health.

Money spent on effective *preventive* medicine does most to keep people healthy; money spent on treatment often does very little.

The Capitation System

In the capitation system of remuneration, the doctor is paid on a head count; that is, on the number of patients to whom he offers medical care. The British Government pays its National Health Service general practitioners in this way. The general practitioner receives $3.60 or so each year for each patient on his practice list.

This system is also fraught with difficulties. Most British general practitioners conduct their practices from premises they either rent or own, and most of them now work in partnership with one or more other doctors. People in the doctor's neighborhood may join his list or the lists of his rivals. To make a reasonable living, a doctor must provide an acceptable enough service to entice patients to join his list and to encourage them to stay on it. He is unwise to discourage patients by refusing to give them barbiturates or amphetamines, or by being difficult about signing specious sick certificates.

In many parts of England, there is a shortage of doctors, and rivalry for patients is not great. By providing pleasant and warm premises, and a competent, quick, and efficient service, the doctor only encourages his patients to use him more often. This increases his work load, but does not bring him greater financial reward. Indeed, such an increase in his work eats into his profits. It increases his expenditures for equipment, paper, stamps, secretarial time, auxiliary help, travel mileage, and telephone services. Any small business that can make money for less work done is not likely to be a hive of useful industry. General practice in Britain now nurtures a discouraging atmosphere of unenthusiasm. Even prescription slips are made just large enough for scribbling a few words of referral of problem cases to the outpatient department of the nearest hospital.

The capitation system of payment has the great advantage that it does not actively encourage treatment enthusiasm. On the other hand, it actively discourages general practitioners from developing particular skills. It offers no particular rewards to the doctor for assiduously treating the acutely sick, the elderly, and the chronically handicapped. Such patients often require many home visits. A great deal of the doctor's time and much hard work can be devoted to cases without any comparable financial reward; for the small per capita fee paid for such patients nowhere near covers the cost of providing proper medical care for them.

Encouraging Laziness

Consequently, the acutely sick are usually sent straight to the hospital; and the old and chronically sick are sometimes neglected. Such cases may be unnecessarily herded into impersonal institutions where medical aid and its auxiliary services are more readily available. Many a patient who could really use help from his family doctor often gets very little of it.

We all like to dump our unwanted problems on other people. The cities of medieval Christendom had an un-Christian habit of collecting all their lunatics together and paying sailors to carry them off to somewhere else. Although this custom had the certain advantage of ridding a city of its problem people, it had the equal disadvantage that a shipload of somebody else's lunatics might at any time be delivered to the city gates. In such an event, both cities just wasted money in transportation fees.

A medical degree does not abolish one's capacity to be

lazy. Patients dump their problems on their doctors. And doctors, unless they have a financial incentive for not doing so, often dump both their patients and their patient's problems onto other doctors. A century of squabble between English general practitioners and specialists illustrates this very nicely.

General Practitioner vs. Specialist

Specialists usually work in hospitals, and general practitioners do not. Before the introduction of health insurance schemes, a patient paid his general practitioner each time his doctor treated him. In contrast, many hospitals were supported by voluntary subscription, and did not need to charge patients. The general practitioners, unhappy at seeing their incomes trotting off to hospitals, wrote frequent articles in the *British Medical Journal* complaining that the specialists were taking away their patients. These general practitioners vigorously opposed expansion of the voluntary hospitals in which these specialists worked. But times change.

In 1911, the National Health Insurance Act made health insurance compulsory for every worker in Britain with an income of under $380 a year. The insured worker attached himself to a general practitioner who was paid 93 cents a year for looking after him, and the worker received the services of his general practitioner free.

No longer paid each time they treated a patient, the general practitioners began to think rather differently about hospitals and specialists. Now they send their insured patients off to both specialists and hospitals. The specialists were soon complaining that they were seeing patients who could be competently treated by their own general practitioners. Because of all their extra work, hospitals had to be bailed out of financial difficulties with Government grants.

With the introduction of the National Health Service, everyone in Britain receives the services of his general practitioner for free. The general practitioner consequently dispatches more patients than ever before off on pilgrimages to outpatient departments. The statistic is now 10 percent of the population of England annually.

Individual doctors vary in the number of patients they refer to hospitals; but a few physicians now send more than 20 percent of all their patients to hospitals every year.

Undoubtedly, a specialist's opinion is sometimes most useful. However, there are real disadvantages for a patient in being sent off to see another doctor. Once two doctors look after a patient, each doctor tends to feel that it is the other man who is really responsible for the case. Both doctors then stop being so. This has been aptly called the "collusion of anonymity" by Michael Balint.

Patient Ping-Pong

Few doctors really want to look after their problem patients. Properly looking after them can prove to be a terrible nuisance. When there is no financial incentive to keep a patient, the general practitioner plays "patient ping-pong" with the hospital doctor. This can be a very dangerous game.

A help-demanding patient is placated with sedatives by his general practitioner until he becomes too toxic and disturbed to stay at home. He is sent to a hospital to be weaned off his pills. After a few months, he is well again and leaves the hospital. He takes himself and his troubles back to his general practitioner. Because sedatives always make him feel better, the doctor gives him some more. If the physician refuses to, the patient changes doctors. Eventually, he gets the pills, swallows them till he gets toxic, and then, six months later, is back in the hospital again. So it goes on. The ping-pong ends when the patient takes too many tablets and is sent to the morgue. No one stops this lethal game because no *one* person is actually playing it.

Under the capitation system of payment, doctors have a financial incentive *to get rid* of their problem patients, and they often do. But then, these general practitioners get bored.

They find they are spending their time writing sick certificates of dubious probity, and prescriptions for treatments of doubtful value. A letter written in 1968 to the *British Medical Journal* expresses what one young doctor thinks of this situation:

> *I qualified 18 months ago; and after registration, there seemed to be two main channels open. General practice I had always regarded as the ideal form of medical practice, but it appeared (and recent experience only confirms this) that if one was to be a general practitioner of integrity with decent premises and facilities, refusing to sign "sick lines" or give prescriptions except when strictly indicated, one was going to lose both money and patients. One was also going to lose most of one's seriously ill patients to hospital service.*

In the middle 1960s, these demoralized British general practitioners threatened to resign from the National Health Service. The British Government then agreed upon a "Charter for the Family Doctor Service." This charter provides grants for improvement of the doctor's premises, subsidies toward paying the salaries of his ancillary helpers, and an increase in the per capita payment for elderly patients.

The Family Doctor's Charter has at least done something to improve the working conditions of general practitioners. But many of these doctors continue to find the capitation system of payment unsatisfactory. They would prefer to be paid for work they do, rather than for work they are *supposed* to do. If, for instance, an American doctor has to make an emergency visit in the middle of his dinner, it is at least some consolation for him to know that his being inconvenienced will help pay for his children's vacations. In the capitation system of payment, such a visit only adds to the doctor's already mounting expenses.

The Fee-for-Service System

The fee-for-service method of payment, because it provides a financial reward for each item of work that the doctor does, removes some difficulties. The snag is that it is difficult to itemize the services of medical practice. It is equally impossible to know if the work itemized actually needed to be done.

One doctor sees a patient with a lengthy story of serious illness. He takes a full history, makes a thorough physical examination, and arranges for the necessary examinations and the treatment regime. A second doctor sees a man who fusses about his health. He quickly takes the patient's blood pressure, looks serious, and prescribes some tablets. Though the first doctor spends more time and does more useful work, both receive the same fee.

Encouraging Crookery

The fee-for-service method of payment requires an army of clerks and bushels of paperwork. It also turns doctors into crooks. It is so easy for the second doctor of our example to suggest that the worried patient should come again. The worried patient is grateful for attention which he does not even have to pay for. The doctor can always check the patient's blood pressure again to make sure that it is still normal. He can prescribe a few tranquilizers, and tell his patient that everything is all right. The doctor is "reassuring his patient." He is also making easy money.

Payment by fee for service turns out to have all the disadvantages of private payment and few of its advantages. Doctors provide treatments galore. It is the system used in West Germany and in Ontario, Canada. Of all the systems of paying doctors, it probably rockets the cost of medical care the most.

In 1971, Bert Lawrence, a former Minister of Health for Ontario, Canada's richest province, commented lugubriously during his first week in office that if the cost of health care in Ontario continued to rise at its present rate, by the year 2000, it would absorb the total gross product of the province.

Quite clearly, many Ontario doctors are taking their government for a ride. One doctor claimed fees for seeing the same 50 patients every day for a month for the treatment of obesity. Some Ontario doctors are said to be charging the government $350,000 a year for the services that they render to their patients.

Even with fee-for-service payment, the very handicapped patients, who perhaps need medical and social care more than the rest of us, still seem to come out badly. Ontario doctors are so busy treating middle-class housewives with Valium and sympathy that they have no time left over to attend to the more complicated requirements of the handicapped.

France and New Zealand also use fee-for-service to pay their general practitioners, but they incorporate in their systems an "offset payment" which is made by the patient. The patient pays the doctor for his services. He is then reimbursed by the health insurance fund, either a specific sum of money or a percentage of the fee. The patient is thus given both a financial interest in the honesty of his doctor, and discouragement from using the medical services unwarrantedly. The system involves many time-consuming small financial transactions, as well as an army of clerks and reams of paperwork.

The Salary System

A regular salary is the simplest way to pay doctors, but it has the disadvantage that the doctor's income remains the same whether he works hard or not. Britain uses this system to pay the hospital doctors who work in the National Health Service; the United States uses this system to pay those doctors who work in government-run hospitals. The Eastern European Communist countries use this system to pay their general practitioners.

Such a payment system is successful when doctors have a set task to perform and a limited number of patients for whom to care. In a more nebulous situation, the doctor becomes just an employee in a vast organization. Direct responsibility for overall management is removed from his hands. If there are still patients to be seen at the end of the day, then this is not his fault; the government should employ more doctors. This is tough on the patients who are still waiting to be seen.

In the Eastern European Communist countries, a free general practitioner service is provided at polyclinics, around which most of the medical care revolves. Each polyclinic is responsible either for a neighborhood, a factory, or a professional group. Much emphasis is placed on preventive medicine. Most treatment is handled on an outpatient basis, but a well-organized system of hospitals exists to which those patients who require hospital care can be referred. Patients are not given a choice of doctor; but if a patient is dissatisfied with the one he has at his own polyclinic, he can, on payment of a small fee, consult a doctor at another clinic.

Encouraging a Black Market

Communist medicine is by no means free from difficulties. Patients complain that the polyclinic doctors are too rushed to spend enough time with them. Doctors complain of the volumes of paperwork that the state requires. The doctors, compared to those in Western countries, are poorly paid. Their salaries are equivalent to those of skilled manual workers and to truck drivers. About 70 percent of all Soviet doctors are women. Doctors in these countries often accept illicit payments from their patients; in Hungary, these are called "tips," and in Poland, "black surgery fees."

Perhaps because of a person's readiness to pay for a little extra personal attention from a doctor in whom he has confidence, the Soviet Union is expanding a system of fee-charging medical clinics for consultation and outpatient care. It is even considering fee-charging hospitals.

Doctors are usually reactionaries; in Communist countries, they have remained a suspect profession. Perhaps rather unkindly, they are held responsible for the high sickness absenteeism rate in these countries, and are often accused of helping malingerers and thus sabotaging the economy. The Soviet Union is worried by the decline both in the quality and the quantity of its health workers.

SOURCES

Balint, Michael: *The Doctor, the Patient and the Illness.* London: Pitman Medical Publishing Co. Ltd., 1957.

Beveridge, Sir William: *Social Insurance and Allied Services.* London: Her Majesty's Stationery Office, 1942.

Bureau of Census: *Statistical Abstract of the U.S.A.* Washington, D. C.: Government Printing Office, 1971.

British Medical Association, Advisory Panel: *Health Services Financing.* London: British Medical Association, 1970.

Champion Expanding Encyclopaedia of Mortuary Practice. No. 361. Oct. 1965. Servicing and Research Dept., The Champion Co., Springfield, Ohio.

Cruckshank, Margaret: "America's Unhealthy Twins." *British Medical Journal,* 1 159 (1969).

Davis, Michael M.: *Medical Care for Tomorrow.* New York: Harper Brothers, 1955.

Encyclopaedia Britannica: "Bismarck."

Ehrenreich, Barbara and John: *The American Health Empire. A Report from Health PAC.* New York: Vintage Books, 1970.

Forsyth, G., and Logan R.: *Gateway or Dividing Line? A Study of Hospital Out-Patients in the 1960's.* London: Oxford University Press, 1968.

Foucault, Michel: *Madness and Civilization: A History of Insanity in the Age of Reason.* Tr. Richard Howard. Toronto: New American Library of Canada, 1967.

Horder, J., and Horder, E.: "Illness in General Practice." *Practitioner,* 173 177 (1954).

Junker, Howard: "Not Gone But Frozen." *Nation,* 206 504 (1968).

Kramer, Joel R.: "Medical Care; as Costs Soar, Support Grows for Major Reform." *Science,* 166 1126 (1969).

Lawrence, Hon. A. R. B.: Symposium on Health Care. Seneca College. Toronto, March 4, 1971. (Economic Council of Canada: Seventh Annual Review: Patterns of Growth. Ottawa: Queen's Printer, 1970).

Levy, Herman: *National Health Insurance: A Critical Study.*

London: Cambridge University Press, 1944.

Lindsey, Almont: *Socialized Medicine in England and Wales.* Chapel Hill: University of North Carolina Press, 1962.

Logan, W. P. D., and Brooke, E. M.: *The Survey of Sickness.* (General Register Office. Studies on Medical and Population Subjects. No. 12.) London: Her Majesty's Stationery Office.

Luk and Tardov in an article in *Lituraturnava Gazeta,* quoted in *The Times* (London), Dec. 10, 1966.

Ministry of Health: *Annual Reports for the Years 1965, 1966 and 1967.* London: Her Majesty's Stationery Office.

Pearce, H. H., and Crocker, L. H.: *The Peckham Experiment. A Study in the Living Structure of Society.* London: George Allen and Unwin, 1943.

Revesz, Laszlo, and Pommor, Hans Jorg: *Der Arzt in Sowjetreich.* Bern: Schweizerisches Ost-Institut, 1965.

Saxton, G. D.: "Annual Meeting of the Canadian Tuberculosis and Respiratory Disease Association." In *Toronto Daily Star,* June 1, 1971.

Schecter, Jerold: "The State of Soviet Medicine." *Time* magazine (Canadian Edition), Oct. 5, 1970.

Sigerst, Henry C.: *On the Sociology of Medicine.* New York: MD Publications, 1960.

Taylor, Gordon Rattroy: *The Biological Time Bomb.* New York: World Publishing Co., 1968.

Toronto Daily Star: "Doctor Overbilling Called Intolerable by Lawrence." May 14, 1971.

Wadsworth, M. E. J., Butterfield, W. J. H., and Blaney, R.: *The Bermonsey Health Survey.* In Press. Reported in W. J. H. Butterfield: *Priorities in Medicine.* London: Nuffield Provincial Hospital Trust, 1968.

Womersley, J.: "The Real Reason for Emigration." *British Medical Journal,* 1 251 (1968).

World Health Organization: Preamble to the Constitution of WHO. Geneva: WHO, 1951.

Medical Politics

Family doctors provide the backbone of medical care. The brighter young doctors become specialists.

The political power of the medical profession remains with specialists, where it is vested in the colleges and hospitals to which they belong. And governments devote much more money to hospitals than to general practice.

The British National Health Service spends seven times as much money on its hospitals as it does on its general practitioners. In Britain, everybody still has a general practitioner, but many of these family doctors now send any patient with a problem straight to a hospital outpatient department to be looked after by specialists.

Family Doctors: An Endangered Species

In the big American cities, family doctors hardly exist anymore. If you are ill, you either stay at home until you are better, manage somehow to get to your doctor's office at his hours, or call an ambulance to go to the crowded emergency department of your local hospital. If you are rich, you telephone your specialist, but you have to be clever to know which one to call.

The cardiologist arrives to find your chest pain is not caused by your heart but by your gall bladder. You send for the gastroenterologist, who finds you anemic. He sends you to the hematologist for iron pills. All three specialists require a fee of $50 and up.

Specialists work in hospitals. Hospital admission is often

the simplest way for the specialist to provide a patient with diagnostic and treatment care. Thus, even though a patient does not need to be tucked up in bed for 24 hours a day, he is often admitted to a hospital anyway.

Two British studies sampling patients in acute hospital wards showed that there was no clinical reason for 25 percent of these patients to be in a hospital. In the United States, where for insurance reasons there are financial advantages both for the patient and doctor to have the patient receive his medical care in a hospital, the percentage of patients in hospitals who really shouldn't be there is even higher.

Inevitably, specialist and hospital care is expensive. Most United States hospitals are profit-making organizations. In 1972, the cost of care in these hospitals *averaged* $100 a day. The state-run hospitals of Britain are less expensive; nevertheless, in 1970, the cost for a hospital bed in a ward for the acutely sick averaged $17 a day. In both the U.S. and Britain, the cost of hospital care is going up fast. In the last 20 years, the cost of keeping a patient in a U.S. hospital has increased by nearly 500 percent.

As more patients are treated in hospitals, hospitals grow bigger. This increase in size brings new problems. In a larger organization, communication becomes difficult, and individual responsibilities become more nebulous. Public relations can be maddeningly impersonal and inconsiderate. Many people find being in a large hospital a very trying experience.

Cut-Throat Competition

Large hospitals usually develop serious disagreements among their staff. These conflicts make providing good health care difficult. Professional helpers probably use up all their goodwill in being nice to tiresome patients, for they certainly have little left over for each other. Problems of status, power, and promotion proliferate. Paramedical personnel—often highly trained, bright young psychologists, biochemists, and social workers holding doctorates in their own subjects—are challenging the dominant positions that physicians continue to occupy in the health hierarchy. Medicine is a profession of cutthroat competition, and senior hospital doctors seldom treat their juniors and future rivals with much grace.

Medical Apprenticeship

In the United States, a young doctor's speciality training lasts only four years. The profitable medical market that awaits him at the end of his training makes it easy for the ambitious and energetic to succeed on his own. In Britain, young specialists in training have a greater problem. Their specialty

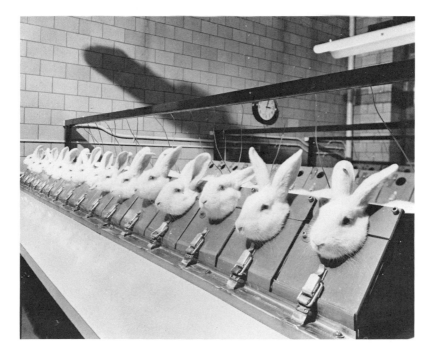

As hospitals grow bigger, many patients feel trapped, like these rabbits. Cost grows higher, and care grows more impersonal.

training lasts 15 years or so. During that time, they are dependent upon the goodwill of their seniors for promotion within the National Health Service.

These junior hospital doctors provide the round-the-clock routine hospital care. They work long hours and are poorly paid, because they are considered to be in training. The senior members of the medical profession have remained rather unconcerned about the plight of their junior colleagues.

The British medical profession demoralizes the would-be specialist by confronting him with a ridiculously difficult examination. The failure rate for doctors taking these tests runs between 80 and 90 percent. This leaves many young doctors feeling professionally hopeless; and of course, less likely to challenge the authority of the establishment. Increasing numbers of young doctors, fed up with doing the work that their seniors are paid to do, and faced with these difficult examinations and an uncertain future, prefer to cross the Atlantic to where the training facilities are more exciting, the pay for junior doctors several times higher, and the hierarchical structure of British medicine a long way off.

Upward and Outward Mobility

It is estimated that between a fifth and a fourth of Britain's young doctors now leave their homeland. In 1968, 378 went to Canada. Canada, the third richest nation in the world, gratefully calculates that she imports $110 million worth of British doctors a year. Britain, in turn, imports doctors from even poorer countries. Half of the junior hospital doctors in hospitals are now from overseas. These doctors, for the most part, take those jobs which, because of the poor pay, the long hours, and the poor prospects for promotion, are eschewed by their colleagues.

The exodus of expensively trained doctors from poorer to richer countries is a loss that the poorer countries can ill afford to sustain. Is it too cynical to conjecture, however, that the governments of these countries are relieved to see their young doctors go to wealthier countries where their expensive habits of treatment can more easily be afforded?

Bucking for Promotion

Just as there is no satisfactory way to pay doctors, there is also no entirely satisfactory way to promote them within the hierarchy of a large State health service. Clinical competence, usefulness to patients, and a capacity for hard work are certainly not the only criteria used in selecting doctors for promotion. Compliance to the wishes of their seniors, and a long list of research publications are equally important. Compliance builds up a conservative hierarchy, resistant to change. Selection by research publications is, on the surface, a sensible manner of rating excellence; nevertheless, it is a system that seems to obscure rather than brighten the light of science.

Research publications on medical subjects are now published at the rate of one every 23 seconds. Since no one is interested in negative findings, every journal editor selects papers with positive findings—papers which show, for instance, that a new cure works better than an old one. Medical science is thus made to appear much more serviceable than it really is. Publishing for promotion exchanges the mask of the witch doctor for that of the scientist; but the patient continues to be hoaxed, and not infrequently harmed, by enthusiastic use of some new medical technique.

SOURCES

British Medical Journal: "Unrest Among Hospital Doctors." **2** 836 (1965).

Combie, D. C., and Cross, K. W.: *Medical Press,* **242** 316 and 340 (1959).

Department of Health and Social Security: *Annual Report for the Year 1970.* London: Her Majesty's Stationery Office, 1971.

Forsyth, G., and Logan, R. F. L.: *The Demand for Medical Care.* London: Oxford University Press, 1960.

Ministry of Health, National Health Service. Circular H. M. (67) 26.

Robinson, Kenneth: Reported in: "Questions in the Commons." *British Medical Journal,* 1 525 (1968).

Royal Commission on Medical Education 1965–68. *Report.* London: Her Majesty's Stationery Office, 1968.

Toronto Daily Star: "U.K.'s 19,000 Doctors Generally Contented to Be Under Medicare." Special Report, Nov. 11, 1970.

The Politics of Patients

For all sorts of reasons, the deliverers of health care do not deliver health very effectively. On the other hand, neither do the targets—you and I—consume it very sensibly.

Four kinds of patients can be delineated: (1) the competent sick; (2) the incompetent sick; (3) the unknowing sick; and (4) the treatment enthusiasts.

The "competent sick" are the good patients of medical practice. They are sick but would rather be well. Before they became sick, they took proper and sensible care to remain healthy. When they are sick, they use their own initiative and the medical help available to recover as quickly as possible. If all patients were like them, the delivery of health care would indeed be much simpler.

The "incompetent sick" are those who are unable to obtain for themselves adequate medical help. The mentally and physically handicapped and the elderly comprise the bulk of this sad group. Supported by a small old age or disability pension, these "hidden sick" eke out their often undernourished and socially isolated lives. No just society can afford to ignore their needs, but for them, the help-providing resources are always overloaded. The incompetent sick are usually forgotten.

The "unknowing sick" are those who are ill but do not know it. In order to discover symptomless illnesses, medical screening programs are being more widely used. Mass x-ray has certainly proved useful.

The Kaiser Permanente Prepaid Medical Group Practice provides care for 2 million people. It has devised computerized and partly automated screening programs that enable at least some serious illnesses to be diagnosed in their early stages. And diagnosing a serious disease at a time when it can still be successfully treated is second in usefulness only to the prevention of the disease in the first place.

The Treatment Enthusiasts

The fourth group is the "treatment enthusiasts," those who devoutly believe in doctors and in treatments.

Ever since the earliest medicine man first waved his wand, doctors have been extolling the virtues of their cures. The modern doctor now has something very real to talk about. It is hardly surprising that some of us have acquired enormous faith in our doctors, and an inordinate enthusiasm for their

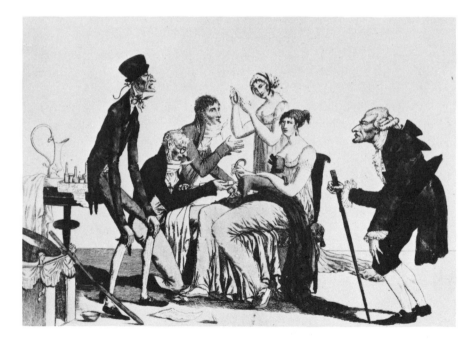

An 18th-century dog receives an enema.

treatments. Nor is it surprising that our demands for treatment have steadily risen.

Whether treatment enthusiasm makes people more healthy and helps them to live longer is not known. It is quite possible

Treatments are love, and man has always shared his favorite treatments with his best friend. A newspaper advertisement from the early years of this century suggests homeopathic treatments for dogs. A present-day Canadian dog has his tonsils removed. Every dog has his day.

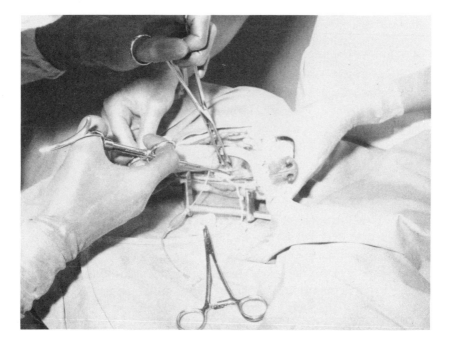

that those who take every minor ailment to the doctor have their serious illnesses diagnosed more quickly.

It is equally possible that they are diagnosed more slowly. Mrs. Jones has visited her doctor twice a month for 20 years. Her smoking eventually catches up with her, and gives her a cancer which makes her cough. Her doctor regards this cough as part of her normal symptom repertoire and sensibly ignores it. Mrs. Jones' cancer is not diagnosed until it is too late to do anything about it.

Mr. Smith is one of the 3 percent or so of us who has not visited the doctor for the past 10 years. The doctor takes his cough more seriously. He refers him for a chest X-ray, and the lung cancer is diagnosed early. Mr. Smith has, at least, a small chance of being cured. But it remains debatable if it is wise to take every minor symptom to the doctor.

Many symptoms that treatment enthusiasts take to the doctor are not minor. In a distressing situation, we all want something useful done. It is most difficult to accept that this may not be possible. Many treatment enthusiasts, when they or their relatives are ill, absolutely insist that their doctors *do* something. Dr. John Fry, a well known London general practitioner, has called these the "gawd sakers"—"for gawd sake, do something." Such patients *force* their doctors into doctoring them. Silly treatments often remain in use because treatment enthusiasts will not let their doctors stop using them, despite the fact the treatment often turns out to be worse than the disease.

The Doctors' Just Dessert

The new health care schemes which make treatment available to everyone covered by them have put doctors in an embarrassing position: everybody now expects to be treated. Doctors who work under these schemes complain that patients come for treatment unnecessarily. But generations of doctors have fostered the virtues of treatment, and patients have come to believe them. Once engendered, treatment enthusiasm does not quickly disappear. Like religion and good table manners, it is handed on by conscientious parents to their children.

Treatment enthusiasm is here to stay; and doctors are, as it were, now being hanged by their own stethoscopes.

Even in the days when all medicine was private, some doctors tried to discourage unrealistic dependence of their patients upon them. Sir William Gull, whose mint-water treatment failed to demonstrate to people their gullibility, would sometimes deliberately refuse to make a second visit so that his patient could discover that recovery was possible without him.

To Charge or Not to Charge

Before the introduction of state health services, it was believed that once doctors were no longer so directly dependent for their income upon patients consulting them, they would not be so tempted into making their patients treatment-dependent. When patients paid for their treatment, a doctor of integrity could suggest that the patient should not waste money on unnecessary visits and useless treatments. The fact that the doctor, by making this suggestion, diminished his own income lent force to his argument. Now that medical services are free, when the doctor suggests that a visit or treatment is unnecessary, the patient suspects that he is trying to wriggle out of doing his duty. It is not the patient's money but somebody else's money that is now being saved.

Charging for medical services means that many sick people cannot afford the medical care they require. Not charging for medical services removes the financial regulator to the use of these services; now these services inundated by treatment enthusiasts become overloaded and inefficient. Charging medical fees discourages the sick from seeking treatment early enough when treatment might be useful; but elimination of the fee, by increasing every doctor's work load, proves as much of a barrier to early care as the medical fee did before health programs were introduced.

Some patients, because they are anxious about themselves, repeatedly have their symptoms investigated by one doctor after another. Other patients manage to book an extraordinary number of appointments with different doctors. One middle-aged Canadian woman had herself investigated by 45 physicians. Within a two-and-one-half-year period, she single-handedly cost the Ontario Medicare plan an estimated $75,000.

The high cost of providing unrestricted medical care leaves little. money left over to spend on preventive care that could be more useful.

Rationing Health Care

Health care is expensive. Because new and more complicated medical techniques are continuously being evolved, health care grows more so every day. No government can afford to provide sufficient resources to meet the total demand for health care; such care has to be rationed. It is easy to ration health care and treatment by price. The rich get it; and the poor, on the whole, go without. Patients get the care they can pay for.

When health care and treatment are provided free, ways must be found of controlling the unlimited demands made upon a limited service. Rationing upsets everybody. Hospitals and doctors cannot be given enough money to supply the services they wish to provide, and their patients do not receive the kind of service to which they feel entitled. Everyone gets cross.

Once the services of our family doctors become free, the doctors are unprotected against the demands we make upon them, and they defend themselves. British doctors, like most other people, work an average 40-hour week; but it is difficult to find a doctor in Britain who does not look tired, who does not complain of the latest epidemic of chicken pox, or who is not about to rush off on an urgent call. A slave of the meanest intelligence knows that the only way to find rest from labor is to appear exhausted or to be unavailable. It behooves the doctor to quickly develop needs of his own, so that he can compete with his patients upon more equal terms. No longer is it necessary in Britain to pay one's doctor, but it is often no longer possible to get one. He is either truly worn out or he is too busy being busy.

Hospital Waiting Lists

Those who advocate having all hospitals taken over as government facilities would do well to study the British experience. British hospitals are not always easy to get into. They use waiting lists to ration their resources. On New Year's Eve 1950, 530,534 people in England and Wales were waiting to get into a hospital. After 20 years of the National Health Service, on New Year's Eve 1970, an almost equal number—525,-926—were waiting. When new hospitals provide more beds, the number of patients immediately expands to fill all the beds available.

If waiting lists did not exist, people would be able to get into a hospital whenever they felt like it. Faced with the exigent plea of illness, the hospital doctors would be hard put to keep anyone out, and to provide care for those who truly needed it. Treatment enthusiasts are quite prepared to argue that a cold in the head may turn into pneumonia, and that a cold anyhow deserves a few days of careful nursing in a hospital. If the doctor personally refuses such a request and the patient does, in fact, catch pneumonia, he can certainly expect to be sued. But a defense of "no beds" is pretty unassailable, both to the patient and, if necessary, to a court.

Having put patients on the waiting list, doctors can then choose to let in whom they will. Only the poison swallowers seriously defeat these lists. Since, without treatment, they may die, they have to be admitted; if necessary, extra beds must be found for them.

On the whole, hospital waiting lists are quite an effective way of rationing a government hospital's services. If the would-be patient feels he cannot wait for his turn, he may decide to pay the expenses of a private doctor and a private hospital. But, as a taxpayer, he may at the same time decide to vote out the party in power.

Delivery of health is no easy matter. In spite of the very real advances that medical science has made and the vast amounts of money that governments and individuals now spend on health, no country has yet devised a health system that works effectively. It may well turn out to be easier to deliver a ballistic missile to a hostile continent than it is to deliver effective health care to our own communities.

SOURCES

Department of Health and Social Security: *Annual Report for the Year 1970*. London: Her Majesty's Stationery Office, 1971.

Eimerl, T. S., and Pearson, R. J. C.: "Working Time in General Practice." *British Medical Journal,* 2 1549 (1966).

Feldstein, M. S.: *Economic Analysis For Health Service Efficiency.* Amsterdam: North Holland Publishing Co., 1967.

Garfield, Sidney R.: "The Delivery of Health Care." *Scientific American,* **222** (4) 15 (1970).

————: "Viewpoint: Free Care Concept May Overload U. S. Health Services." *Geriatrics,* **26** (4) 41 (1971).

Hale-White, Sir William: *Great Doctors of the 19th Century.* London: Edward Arnold and Co., 1935.

Lewis, Sir Aubrey: "Medicine and the Affections of the Mind." *British Medical Journal,* 2 1549 (1963).

Ministry of Health: *Annual Report for the Year 1950.* London: Her Majesty's Stationery Office, 1951.

Powell, J. Enoch: *A New Look at Medicine and Politics.* London: Pitman's Medical Publishing Co., Ltd., 1966.

The Right to Survive

Abide with me; fast falls the eventide;
The darkness deepens; Lord, with me abide;
When other helpers fail, and comforts flee,
Help of the helpless, O, abide with me.
Swift to its close ebbs out life's little day;
Earth's joys grow dim, its glories pass away;
Change and decay in all around I see;
O Thou, who changest not, abide with me.

HENRY FRANCIS LYTE

An unkind saying has it that "God gets only the women that men don't want." Certainly the Church once provided a haven for the lonely, the misfit, and the inadequate. Our universe expands, and the problems of our world increase. Few of us do not sometimes feel like a small child lost in a large city. We wonder why we are here, where we are going, and what will become of us. Most of us would like to hold the hand of somebody who knows. Only God used to hold out that kind hand—now doctors hold out theirs.

Many people place more faith in the medical profession than in God, and doctors often collude by supporting the hopeful belief that the medical profession can and will provide the answers to our health and happiness. It is, of course, fun playing God; some doctors fill the part quite nicely. But very serious health problems now face mankind.

The new system of health care is concerned with our social right to be looked after, a subject for endless discussion and controversy. We have no biological right to survive unless we are adaptable enough to do so.

The Specter of Extinction

Encumbered by our ever increasing numbers, and imprisoned by the exigencies of our own technology, it becomes increasingly difficult for us to adapt to the world in which we live. Existence is perilous. In the long course of evolution, 98 percent of all animal and plant species that have inhabited this earth have slipped into extinction. In the past 400 years, about 170 known species of animals have become extinct due to man's burgeoning progress. Many biologists believe that our own existence now stands in peril.

Two amorous houseflies starting in the spring could theoretically produce enough descendants by the fall to cover the world 47 feet deep in flies. But the world does not become draped with a mantle of houseflies; hungry birds and a million other housefly disasters insure that, in the long run, each parent fly is succeeded by only one fly.

A Limit to Growth

Living matter, when given the right conditions, will continue to grow indefinitely. In the finite conditions of our planet, such unlimited growth is obviously not possible. Lack of food or the accumulated waste products of living matter inevitably curtail such growth. But living things in their many forms have usually evolved ways of limiting their growth—long before they are starved by lack of food, or poisoned by their own putrescence. Closest to home, the living cells of our own bodies respond to little-understood mechanisms that limit their increase in numbers. Cancer is a breakdown of this mechanism. Individual cells no longer respond to control, and be-

come rampant in their multiplication. They kill both themselves and us.

A few species of animals, when they are comfortably surrounded by food, do, in fact, just continue to multiply until
they eat themselves out of existence. The whole population
then starves to death. When the food supply is replenished,
the area is recolonized by individuals of the same kind from
other areas, and the whole process starts again. Tent caterpillars, which sometimes festoon the trees of North America
for miles, "cycle" their populations in this way.

But most animal species have managed to iron out, at
least to some extent, such catastrophic fluctuations in their
numbers. Some live in tranquil equilibrium with their para-
sites and predators. Some have developed chemical control
of their numbers. For instance, some flour beetles secrete a
gas that both dampens their sex interests and is lethal to their
larvae. The more dense the bettle population, the more dense
the unaphrodisiacal lethal gas.

Many animal species have evolved capitalistic patterns of
behavior that insure that only the property owners breed. A
robin must find a territory and defend it before any female
will even consider him. Whatever the unpropertied may think
of such landed privilege, it does, at least, help to make sure
there will be sufficient worms to feed the next generation of
robins.

Although some mammals have had success in diminishing
the size of their population cycles, many others, from voles to
caribou, still have broad fluctuations in population. The non-
cyclic mammal remains the exception rather than the rule.
Biologists have made careful studies of the rise and fall of the
population of the Minnesotan jack rabbit. Jack rabbits cycle
their populations every 10 years. At their population peaks,
the rabbits get "shock disease" that causes vast numbers of
them to die off.

The General Adaptive Syndrome

The cause of shock disease was a biological mystery until 1948, when Hans Selye published his famous paper on the "general adaptive syndrome." This syndrome occurs in an animal when it is exposed to continuous stress. Its adrenal glands enlarge and secrete increasingly large amounts of adrenocortical hormones. These hormones help the animal to survive the stressful situation. If the stress continues long enough, the adrenal glands become exhausted, and the secretion of adrenocortical hormones fails. The animal goes into a state of shock and dies.

Hans Selye's general adaptive syndrome was once thought to provide the answer to the cause of some serious human diseases such as rheumatoid arthritis and ulcerative colitis, which then became regarded as diseases of stress. Psychiatrists in the 1950s were delighted to find that the mind could cause such physical havoc. It put a very large feather in their caps, and helped them to establish themselves in general hospitals.

Though psychiatrists have kept their feather, few doctors now believe that stress or the general adaptive syndrome causes these diseases. However, the general adaptive syndrome did provide the answer to the population fluctuation of jack rabbits.

The population crashes of mammals are not as total as those of the tent caterpillar. Some jack rabbits, for instance, survive. Those that do so, return to the proverbial habits of rabbits with apparent ease of mind. Their population cycle starts all over again.

Overcrowding

Overcrowding distresses many animals. Under such conditions, protective parental behavior deteriorates. Even that baby-bringer to coy families, the white stork, will deliberately kill and eat its own chicks when its nesting sites have become too crowded. Nor are storks alone in such behavior. Animals as different as mice and lions, when their numbers exceed the limits that their environment can carry, neglect, kill, and often eat their own young.

Wolves have exemplary success in keeping the size of

their populations constant. When wolves are shot or poisoned by man, more females litter; from each litter, more puppies survive. Nearly half of a wolf population must be killed each year before their numbers are reduced. The dominant females of these socially well-structured lupine societies apparently control the breeding of their subordinates by letting them have puppies only when such are needed to replace the wolves that have died or have been killed. Without such a mechanism, hungry wolves would soon exterminate all those animals upon which they depend for their food. Then there would be no wolves.

Prehistoric hunters and food gatherers maintained an infinitesimally low population-growth rate, probably by using some such similar social mechanisms to limit numbers. In present-day primitive societies, all sorts of social customs, from sexual taboos to infanticide and head hunting, serve to maintain the size, and therefore the stability, of these societies.

But most societies have long since outgrown such tribal organization. Most of us now live in big cities. Do we do well in them? "Of all animals, men are the leasted fitted to live in herds," wrote Rousseau, as he hankered after the noble savage. But Rousseau's knowledge of biology was pretty flimsy: in comparison to other mammals, modern man seems remarkably unaffected by overcrowded conditions. Indeed, we seem to prefer to congregate in the concrete jungles of our large cities.

Nevertheless, scientists do not really know if crowded living conditions are detrimental to good behavior. René Spitz, a world authority on human behavior, suggests that the quality of human mothering deteriorates in crowded conditions. Like other mammals in an unsatisfactory environment, human beings can make deplorable parents. Seoul, the poor and overcrowded capital of Korea, leads the world with its figures for child abandonment: 105 children are abandoned each month, more than half of them to die in the orphanages in which they are placed.

The Battered-Child Syndrome

Seoul is no worse than poverty-stricken 18th- and 19th-century Europe. Of the 500,000 babies abandoned between 1728 and 1757 to the care of English parish workhouses, more than 60 percent died before the age of two. Nor is our present behavior vis-à-vis our children very laudable. Within the past few years, on both sides of the Atlantic, there has been a large increase in the numbers of reported cases of parents injuring their young. Probably such injuries have always been quite common, but doctors were too naive to realize that the severe injuries they were seeing in children were often inflicted by the parents themselves.

In 1946, an American radiologist reported that X-rays of children with head injuries not infrequently showed multiple fractures of the limbs in various stages of healing. After other radiologists confirmed this report, it began to be suspected that these repeated injuries were the result of parental ill treatment. In 1962, an American pediatrician and his co-workers, reporting on 749 cases of babies and children who had been seriously injured or killed by their parents, coined the term "the battered-child syndrome" to describe their findings. They concluded that parental physical abuse was a major cause of death and maiming in American children. Since then, laws have been passed in all 50 states requiring that cases of child abuse be reported.

In 1967 and 1968, the Children's Bureau of the Department of Health, Education, and Welfare conducted a nationwide study of children who were reported to have received parent-inflicted injuries. In these two years, 12,600 children were found to have received injuries of varying severity. Of these children, 580 were left with permanent damage, and 428 died of their injuries. It is estimated that about 10,000 cases of the battered-child syndrome occur in the United States each year.

The first case of the battered-child syndrome in the United Kingdom was reported in 1963. A British Government report

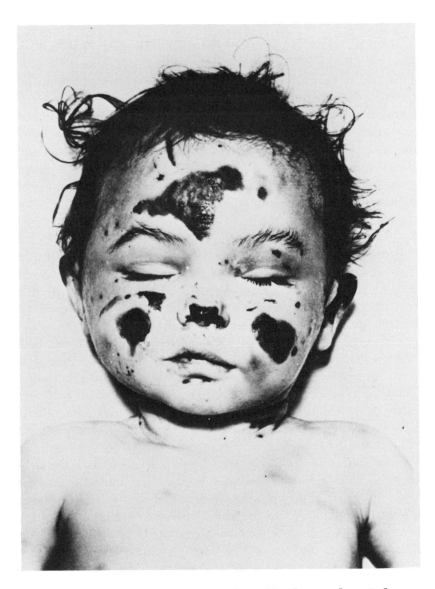

This child died from injuries inflicted by his mother. Baby battering occurs in all classes of society, but it is most prevalent in poor families with large numbers of children, many of them unwanted.

published in 1970 estimates that at least 3,000 babies and children are injured or seriously deprived by their parents each year, and that at least 40 babies, aged less than one year, die through such injury.

Baby battering occurs in all classes of society; but it occurs most often in poor families with large numbers of children. Not infrequently, these babies were unwanted. Affectionate and constructive behavior is learned, so it is hardly surprising that battered babies grow to be disturbed and destructive adults whose unhappy and revengeful behavior is a problem for society to contain. Neither is it surprising that these adults, in their turn, become walloping parents.

It is not known if babies are battered mostly because their parents were themselves treated in this way. Battering, some psychiatrists believe, is a biological response to overcrowding. Other battering takes place because society, with its often rigid rules against abortion, insists that women have babies they do not want. Man is a mammal, and for the human baby as for any other baby mammal, it is probably not safe to be born unwanted into an overcrowded community.

Malthusian Pessimism

Like other members of the animal kingdom, multiplying man has a problem with his numbers. "The human population," asserted the unpopular Thomas Malthus 200 years ago, tends to grow "geometrically," and food supply only "arithmetically." Inevitably, he maintained, the infinite human hopes for happiness must be in vain. Population would increase to the level of subsistence, to be relentlessly held there by war, famine, and ill health. Only contraception, self-restraint, or misery could prevent the inevitable increase in human numbers. Since the Reverend Malthus regarded contraception as a vice and, sensibly, self-restraint as impractical, only misery and poverty remained as man's inescapable lot.

This dismal prospect for mankind was liked only by hardheaded 19th-century industrialists. Such an uncompromising' theory of the human condition amply justified their refusal to raise the pitifully low wages with which they rewarded their workers.

Times changed, and Malthusian pessimism was forgotten. Vast stretches of arable lands were opened up in America and Australia, and technology seemed capable of working miracles. Unquestionably, ever since men stopped being hunters and food gatherers and settled down to become respectable agriculturalists, technical achievements have been astounding.

We have made our grain grow bigger and our animals more sturdy. We control most of the diseases that once ravaged our animals, our plants, and ourselves. We can fix the

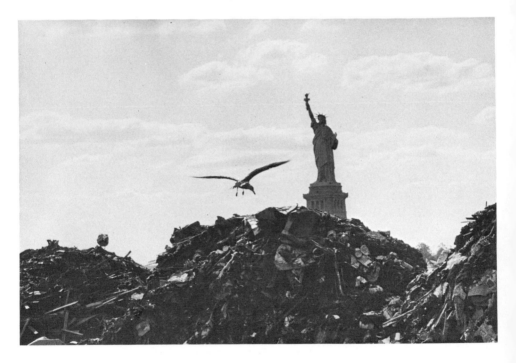

The effluent of affluence. The Statue of Liberty salutes a garbage barge traveling out to sea. How much liberty can we take with the sea before we poison it?

nitrogen in the air to make artificial fertilizers. We can make our lands burgeon with food, and we can transport that food rapidly around the world. Everywhere machines replace human toil. Even computers help in the feeding of our growing numbers. In the face of such achievement, it is not surprising that it has become customary to thumb one's nose to the hare-lipped Reverend Malthus.

But with the recent ecology-mindedness, it is now anxiously asked, "Will Malthus prove to be right?"

The Ecological Prognosis

Let us look at geometrical or, as it is now more correctly called, exponential expansion. Early man doubled the size of his population every 22,000 years or so. The world population rose from about 5 million in 6,000 B.C. to about 500 million in A.D. 1650. By 1850, it was 1 billion. It rose to 2 billion in 1930; and to 3 billion in 1960. Today, the world population is more than 3.5 billion. At the present rate of increase, world population will grow to 7 billion by the end of this century.

If the world population continues to increase at its present rate, in 2,000 to 3,000 years there will be so many people in the world that they would weigh more than the world itself. Long before this, we would be packed together like sardines. Sardines in a can can be eaten, but can they eat?

Playing Dirty

The fully fed nations of the world maintain their well stocked supermarkets and the coziness of their living standards by the prowess of their industrial techniques. In doing so, they use up more than their fair share of strictly limited fossil fuels and raw materials. The United States, with 6 percent of the world's population, uses 30 percent of the world's resources. The rich nations are turning the world into a garbage dump.

High-yield agriculture, industrial processes, car engines,

and household rubbish overload and poison the natural waste disposal properties of our ecosystem. Fertilizers drain from farmlands into rivers and lakes. The algae grow faster. The overgrowth of algae excludes sunlight from the water, and the algae die and putrefy. This uses up the oxygen in the water, and the fish also die. Lakes and rivers die along with their dead fish.

Farmers do not want insects to eat their crops. Each year, they use over 100 million pounds of pesticides to discourage these myriads of munching mandibles. Some of these

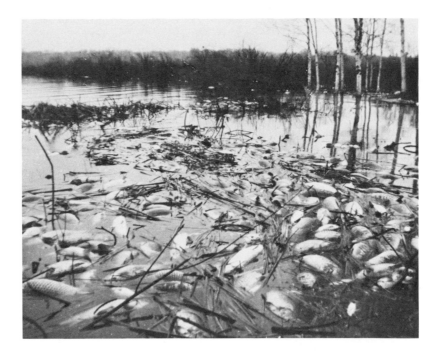

Dead fish float on our polluted waters. Rivers and lakes die, too, as fertilizers drain in from the farmlands and feed the algae. The algae grow so numerous that they soon exclude sunlight from the water. They die and putrefy, using up the oxygen in the water. When the oxygen goes so do the living things in the water.

pesticides, like long-lasting DDT, are now firmly established in a tangle of food chains, and so poison birds and fish. Perhaps, they will soon be poisoning us, too.

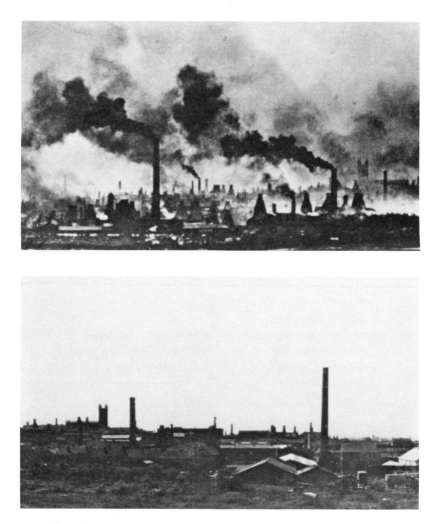

England's Stoke-on-Trent makes pottery, and once also made dirt. These two photographs, taken in 1910 and 1969, illustrate the effectiveness of pollution control. It is better to treat chimneys than damaged lungs.

Thermal pollution from nuclear power stations imperils the rich marine life of the world's estuaries. Mercury and other poisons from industrial waste and untreated sewage pour out into the rivers of the world. Already, swordfish has been banned by the United States as food—its mercury concentration is a hazard to health.

Dead rivers carry death to the oceans, and these already have their own killers. The Torrey Canyon tanker disaster that aroused many people's indignation spilled 100,000 tons of oil onto the British coast. But 300,000 tons of oil are spilled by ships and oil rigs into the oceans every year. Crude oil contains substances toxic to sea life. The Mediterranean now rushes toward total pollution. Jacques-Yves Cousteau reports that overfishing and pollution in the past 20 years have reduced all marine life by 40 percent. Soon, we will not have fish on Fridays.

We load our atmosphere with dirt. Plants make the life-giving oxygen of our atmosphere. The vegetation of the United States can now supply only 60 percent of the oxygen that the country uses each year for the combustion of fossil fuels. Each year, America pours 72 million tons of toxic carbon monoxide into the air.

Since the middle of the 19th century, the amount of carbon dioxide in the atmosphere has been steadily rising. Carbon dioxide lets sunlight through, but traps thermal radiation from the earth. The increased carbon dioxide in the atmosphere makes the earth hotter; but the dust we pump into the atmosphere traps sunlight and makes the world colder. If carbon dioxide and dust pollution get out of balance, will we survive the change in climate? Will our fat new rice and wheat and maize still grow?

Not only will the supply of fossil fuels, and of many of the raw materials upon which our present high level of industrialization depends, inevitably run out—only the exact time remains in some doubt—but it is possible that the waste products of our society will, before then, poison the very world upon which our life depends.

Closing Our Eyes to the Future

Nobody wants to go hungry. Only by industrialization can the underfed nations of the world feed themselves. These nations also want factory chimneys, pesticides, and fertilizers.

Nobody wants to be poor. We who live in an industrial society want our jobs and our profits. The local mill pours mercury into the lake. This hurts everybody just a little. Close the mill down, and the owners lose their profits and the workers lose their jobs. This hurts a lot. We are all human; and the specter of immediate and personal disaster is worse than the threat of some distant and general catastrophe. Naturally, the mill stays open.

Capitalists and Communists alike pollute the world. We are in a jam, and there is no easy way out.

SOURCES

British Medical Journal: "Battered Babies." 3 667 (1969).

Caffey, John: "Multiple Fractures in the Long Bones of Infants Suffering Chronic Subdural Haematoma." *American Journal of Roentgenology, Radium Therapy and Nuclear Medicine,* 56 163 (1946).

Christian, John J.: "The Adrenal-Pituitary System and Population Cycles in Mammals." *Journal of Mammalogy,* 31 24 (1950).

Coale, Ansley J.: "Man and His Environment." *Science,* 170 132 (1970).

Cole, LaMont C.: "Playing Russian Roulette with Biogeochemical Cycles." In *The Environmental Crisis.* Ed. Harold W. Helfrich. New Haven: Yale University Press, 1970.

Department of Health and Social Security: *Annual Report for the Year 1969.* London: Her Majesty's Stationery Office, 1970.

————: *The Battered Baby.* London: Her Majesty's Stationery Office, 1970.

Ehrlich, Paul R.: "Famine 1975, Fact or Fallacy?" In *The Environmental Crisis.* Ed. Harold W. Helfrich. New Haven: Yale University Press, 1970.

Encyclopaedia Britannica: (1972): "Population."

Gates, David: "Weather Modification in the Service of Mankind: Promise or Peril?" In *The Environmental Crisis.* Ed. Harold W. Helfrich. New Haven: Yale University Press, 1970.

Gil, David G.: *Violence Against Children.* Cambridge: Harvard University Press, 1970.

Green, R. G., Larson, C. L., and Bell, J. F.: "Shock Disease as the Cause of the Periodic Decimation of Snowshoe Hares." *American Journal of Hygiene,* Sect. B 30 83 (1939).

Guttermacher, Alan F.: "Unwanted Pregnancy: A Challenge to Mental Health." *Mental Hygiene,* 51 512 (1967).

Hoagland, Hudson: "Cybernetics of Population Control." In *Human Fertility and Population Problems.* Ed. Roy O. Greep. Cambridge: Schenkman Publishing Co., Inc., 1963.

Howell, Nancy Lee: Office of Population Research, Princeton University; personal communication, 1971.

Kempe, Henry C.; Silverman, Frederick N.; Steele, Brandt F.; Droegemueller, William; and Silver, Henry K.: "The Battered Child Syndrome." *Journal of the American Medical Association,* **181** 17 (1962).

Lake, David C.: *The Life of the Robin.* London: Pelican Books, 1953.

Langer, Wm. L.: "Checks on Population Growth." *Scientific American,* **226** (2) 93 (1972).

Mech, David: *The Wolf. The Ecology and Behavior of an Endangered Species.* New York: Natural History Press, 1970.

National Tuberculosis and Respiratory Diseases Association: *Air Pollution Primer.* New York, 1967.

Oliver, J. E., and Taylor, Audrey: "Five Generations of Ill-Treated Children In One Family Pedigree." *British Journal of Psychiatry,* **119** 473 (1971).

Pimlott, Douglas, H.: "The Life of the Timber Wolf." *Living Wilderness,* **34** (111) 20 (1970).

Selye, Hans: "The General Adaptive Syndrome and the Diseases of Adaption." *Journal of Clinical Endocrinology and Metabolism,* **6** 117 (1946).

Spitz, René A.: "The Derailment of Dialogue: Stimulus Overload, Action Cycles, and the Completion Gradient." *Journal of the American Psychoanalytic Association,* **12** 752 (1964).

Time magazine: "Environment: Issue of the Year" (Canadian Edition). Jan. 4, 1971.

———: "Environment: To Save the Seas" (Canadian Edition). Dec. 28, 1970.

———: "In Memory of Man's Victims" (Canadian Edition). April 26, 1971.

———: "Man Into Superman: The Promise and the Peril of the New Genetics" (Canadian Edition). April 19, 1971.

Young, Gordon: "Pollution: Threat to Man's Only Home." *National Geographic,* **138** 739 (1970).

Wiggins, J. R.: Address to Plenary Session of the United Nations on the Problems of Human Environment. Dec. 3, 1968.

Population Control

We are unable to provide even the bare necessities of life for all the 3.5 billion people alive today. It is inconceivable that we will be able to do so for the 7 billion people who, at the present rate of population increase, will be alive at the end of this century. People will be crowded together in vast metropolises. Even Britain, with one of the world's slowest growth rates, will have another 11 million people packed into its islands.

Calcutta is scheduled to be the world's largest city. Expanding at the rate of 300,000 people a year, by the end of the century it will have a population somewhere between 36 million and 60 million. Yet the deteriorating mental and physical health of people in cities one-hundredth this size is already a matter of deep social concern. Even now, Calcutta cannot afford to construct new sewers, and sewage runs in gutters in the streets.

A Question of Food

Quite clearly, the world is not going to be able to cope unless drastic measures are taken. Many ecologists believe it is too late to prevent world famine in this century. It has perhaps already started. Despite advances in agriculture and increases in national food output, the world's population is increasing faster than its food supplies. Some ecologists predict a catastrophic decline in population to about a third of our present size within the next few decades.

Famine is nothing new in human history. From the days

of the ancient Egyptians when the Nile failed to flood to the present time, the pages of history have been blotched by the devastation of starvation. Hand in hand with war and pestilence, the social degradation that famine causes has stalked our progress. In times of famine, cats, dogs, horses, and rats are all devoured; and soon after that stage, men become cannibals. Men eat their wives; and wives, their husbands. Parents eat their children. When food supplies run out, even well-equipped hospitals cannot save children from starvation.

Animals are usually protected from the disasters of overcrowding by their instinctual behavior patterns. We, the most intelligent of living creatures, have largely escaped from the bondage—and the safety—of instinct. Our bright intelligence

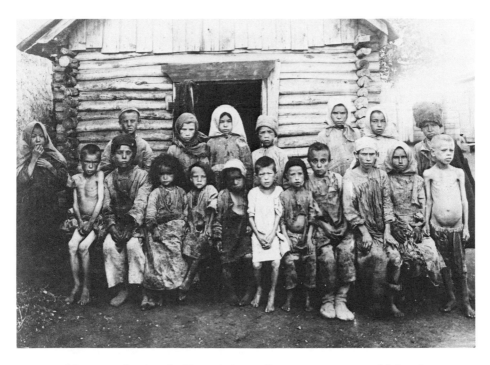

Many ecologists believe it is too late to avert a world famine in this century. For these poor children, it has already started.

allows for the insightful determination of at least some of our behavior. But will our bright intelligence be enough? Will we be bright enough to limit our numbers before we ourselves are plunged into the disaster of social chaos or into the abyss of a cyclic population collapse?

Creatures of Habit

Death control must be balanced by life control. Our attempt to have the first without the second is one of the most flagrant examples ever of wanting to have one's cake and eating it.

Effective life control means the use of both contraception and abortion, and many people object strongly to both. Both these forms of birth control provide tricky theological conundrums for those who choose to be stuck with such puzzles. For all of us, birth control provides the chance to use our sexuality for joy and not for procreation. This notion certainly puts many people into a tizzy of anxiety.

The church, the medical profession, and the law often impose sanctions against the use of contraception and abortion. Many of us stick to our well-worn convictions that sex is evil. We are creatures of habit. We detest change, preferring whenever possible to hold fast to our life-long habits of mind. But the world around us changes fast. Can we afford to remain the same?

Christian theologians have never approved of sex. When, after years of laboratory toil, Paul Ehrlich discovered a spirochaeticide for the treatment of syphilis, the church opposed its use on the grounds that syphilis was a fitting punishment for immorality.

Neither were Christian doctrinaires pleased to have women escape the pains of childbirth. "In pain shall you bring forth children," states the Bible. When chloroform inhalation was found to relieve these pains, its use was vehemently attacked in Britain by both pamphlet and pulpit. Queen Victoria eventually put an end to the furor. Fed up with the pain of six previous deliveries, she requested chloro-

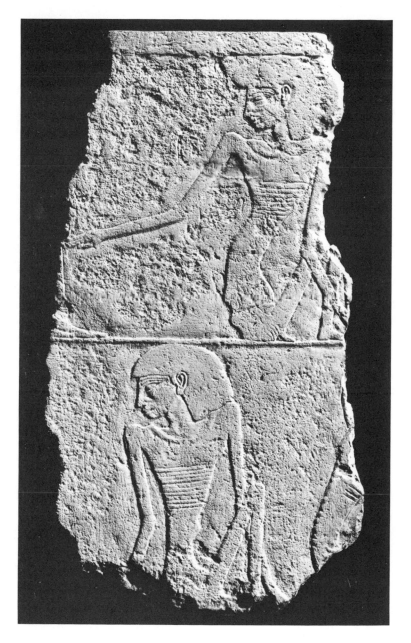

Lean years in ancient Egypt are recalled by this emaciated figure from the pyramid of Ounas, near Gizeh.

form for the birth of Prince Leopold; after that, everyone kept quiet.

Leopards do not change their spots. Faced with the choice of changing its traditional beliefs or of trying to stop the world's head-on collision with disaster, the Catholic Church clings to its beliefs. Let the world look after itself.

Puritanical pessimism demands that sexual enjoyment must lead to discomfort, disease, and disaster. For the Victorians, lovemaking had to end in painful labor, and masturbation in madness. For our Edwardian grandparents, the promiscuous had to catch syphilis. For the United States State Department, homosexuality must end in Communism and corruption. For the psychoanalyst, abortion must end in guilt. For Catholics, copulation must end in children, however unwanted these may be.

Abortion and the Doctors

The medical profession is not much more helpful. Traditionally, abortion has been contrary to its ethics. The Hippocratic Code, which has more or less guided the conduct of doctors for the past 2,300 years, adjures the doctor not to aid women to procure an abortion.

Hippocrates wrote his works a long time ago, and there is considerable doubt as to which part of them he actually wrote. It has been suggested that it was his austere Pythagorean disciples and not Hippocrates himself who wrote the injunction against abortion. Those who believe this point to Hippocrates' recommendation to a dancing girl that she take violent exercise to rid herself of her unwanted foetus.

Abortion was certainly regarded as acceptable practice by most of the ancient world. Plato and Aristotle, the intellectual and moral giants of that world, and Hippocrates' younger contemporaries, both approved of abortion as a sensible method for limiting the otherwise inevitable increase in human numbers. Aristotle even suggested that a woman should be compelled to abort herself after she had borne an allotted number of children.

In spite of the church's tight-lipped disapproval and in spite of the Hippocratic Code, abortion was not made a crime in England until the early 1800s, nor in the United States until about the middle of the century, when each country was in the middle of its Industrial Revolution. Filth, poverty, and sepsis were everywhere.

In those days, being admitted to a hospital for a surgical operation ran a close second in health to being put directly

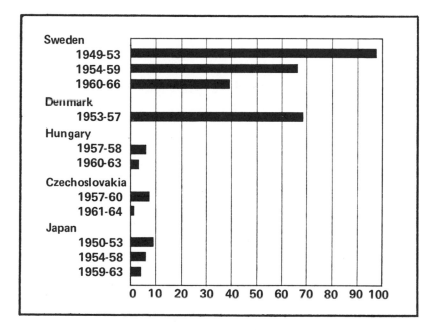

This chart illustrates the mortality ratios per 100,000 abortions in those countries that have liberalized their abortion statutes. The Scandinavian nations have higher death rates than one might otherwise expect simply because their abortion laws have been only partially liberalized. In these countries, abortions are often restricted to women in poor physical health. Also, because Scandinavian officials regularly take several weeks to consider a petition for abortion, many abortions are not performed until the third or fourth month of pregnancy, at which time the chance of death is four times greater.

into the morgue. Before Lister revolutionalized surgery by the use of carbolic antiseptics, so many patients died of septic wounds in the hospital where Lister practiced that new patients were asked to deposit money to cover possible funeral expenses.

The aborted uterus is most vulnerable to infection. In the pre-Listerian industrial squalor of the last century, abortion became a most hazardous operation. It was for health reasons and not for theological reasons that abortion was made illegal.

The all-or-none philosophies with which our forefathers tried to understand themselves and their world required that a body either did or did not have a soul. Nothing in between would do. The Greeks generally believed that the unborn child acquired an "animate" soul some time after conception. Hippocrates put this time at about 30 days for males. Since the Greeks considered women to be not quite so with it, the time was set at about 42 days for females.

Our English forebears, being on the whole more practical than the Greeks, considered that life and the soul did not enter the unborn child until the child first quickened at about midterm. Abortion before quickening was no crime.

The Victorians got themselves hooked on the soul as well as on senna. A headmaster of Eton College preached to his pupils that at the moment of death a man lost weight due to its departure. What got out had to get in, and in their concern the Victorians wanted the soul in as quickly as possible, so they slipped it in with a sperm. At the moment of conception, the ovum became a living being and abortion became murder. The Offences Against the Persons Act of 1861 made even the attempt to procure an abortion punishable by life imprisonment. Only the abortion of a pregnancy that endangered the life of the mother remained permissible.

The Bourne Case

In 1938, a 14-year-old English girl was raped by three troopers of the Royal Horse guards in the stables of Whitehall. Alec Bourne, a brave and distinguished gynecologist, admitted he aborted her. He was tried as a criminal. Bourne was eventually acquitted—but not on the ground that it was proper to terminate the pregnancy of a 14-year-old girl who did not wish to bear a child that was fathered upon her by force. Rather, he was acquitted on the legal quibble that a continuation of the pregnancy would have endangered her health—her mental health. After this cause célèbre, it was permissible in Britain to abort a woman for the protection of her mental health.

We live in a "sick-making society." Bourne's legal precedent has managed to put yet another illness into Pandora's overcrowded box. In England, any intelligent woman with an unwanted pregnancy just has to throw hysterics and threaten suicide, and almost certainly two doctors will be prepared to certify that her mental health will be damaged by the continuation of her pregnancy. She gets her abortion. The moral of this is: threaten to be sick, feeble, and incompetent, and you can usually make professional helpers do what you want them to.

Recent Developments

In 1967, the English Abortion Act carried this precedent into law. It also made abortion lawful if there is a substantial risk that the child will be born seriously handicapped, or if the continuation of the pregnancy threatens the well-being of the mother's already existing children. This last phrase has become known as the "social clause." The social clause in England's abortion law has done something to protect the children of large and underprivileged families from being battered by their exhausted and reluctant parents. But note that the British Medical Association and the Royal College of Obstetricians and Gynecologists objected strongly to the social clause.

In 1970, New York State almost abolished its restrictive abortion laws. Abortion was made legal up to the 24th week of pregnancy on the request of the mother; not even her husband had to be consulted. By June, 1970, four other states had virtually repealed all statutes regulating abortion, and 17 other states had reformed their abortion laws. Only four states retained their old codes. In 1973, the U.S. Supreme Court overruled all state laws that prohibit or restrict a woman's right to obtain an abortion during her first three months of pregnancy. For the first three months the decision to have an abortion lies with the woman and her doctor. The states' interests are not "compelling" enough to warrant any interference.

Abortion was once a dangerous operation; there were good reasons for discouraging it. But once-upon-a-time sensible health regulations often end up as tiresome moral injunctions. Abortion is now safer than having a baby. In Czechoslovakia and Hungary where abortions are performed in state clinics, the death rate is as low as three per 100,000 operations. By contrast, 20 of every 100,000 American women die from the complications of childbirth.

Of all the many sorts of human relationships, the helper-helpee relationship is the most prone to disaster. Priests have burned parishioners for the good of their souls, and doctors have too often imposed their own moral—not just medical—judgments on their patients. Is it best for women to have children they do not want, and for all of us to have so many people in this world that there will be a disaster? These questions are for all of us to decide, and not just for the gynecologists and the priests.

Contraception

Throughout history, people have used contraceptives. An early Egyptian papyrus recommends that a paste of crocodile dung and honey be inserted in the vagina before intercourse. Contraceptives have become, if not more efficient, at least less messy. But none of them have proved to be the complete answer to the erstwhile maiden's prayer, or even to that of the

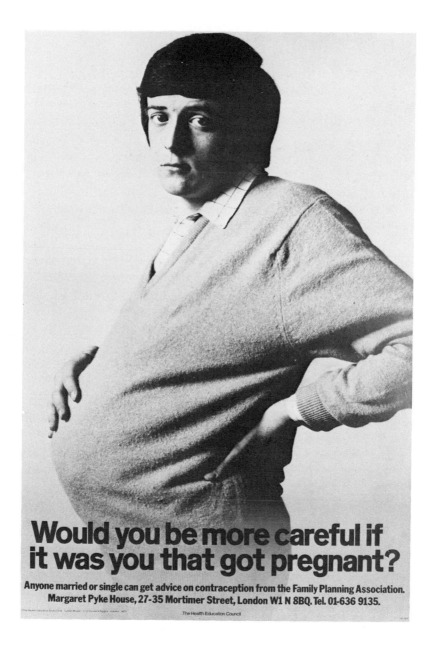

Would you be more careful if it was you that got pregnant?

Anyone married or single can get advice on contraception from the Family Planning Association. Margaret Pyke House, 27-35 Mortimer Street, London W1 N 8BQ. Tel. 01-636 9135.

The Health Education Council

This poster was issued by the Health Education Council of Great Britain in 1970, and has been published—with variations in native dress—in 24 countries.

decently married woman. Contrary to usual belief, it is the latter who most often finds herself with an unwanted pregnancy.

Only a fetishist can really like a condom. Intrauterine devices give tummy cramps. Diaphragms require unnatural premeditation, and they get left behind on vacations. "The Pill" gives its users the creeps each time a newspaper headlines that "The Pill Kills Another Woman."

Since many of us spend much of our lives being wise only after the event, unwanted pregnancies, like other disasters, will inevitably occur. Because reliable contraceptives are not always safe, and safe contraceptives are not always reliable, even the most sensible and far-sighted women continue to find themselves in trouble. Abortion is a far from perfect way of providing family planning, but it is effective.

The Japanese Eugenics Act of 1948 allows abortion to be obtained at the request of the mother. The Soviet Union, having blown hot and cold in its attitude, made abortion more freely available again in 1958, and the Communist East European states soon followed suit. Unlike the rest of the world, Japan and the Communist European countries rapidly reduced their birth rates.

The demand for abortion is high. Japan has a population of nearly 100 million. In 1955, Japanese doctors legally aborted 1,170,000 pregnant women. Contraceptives then became popular, and by 1967, the annual number of abortions had fallen to 748,000. Unfortunately, the statistician's job is never easy; and doctors, like everyone else, are not always honest. It is suspected that Japanese doctors, for income tax reasons, did not report all their abortions. Even the recorded figures make the 80,000 legal·abortions performed in England and Wales in 1970 seem meager.

Although the Japanese abortion rates are high, the rates in many countries with strong scruples against this operation are not much different. In countries where even contraception is discouraged, women avoid having unwanted children by having illegal abortions instead. Abortion is the foremost

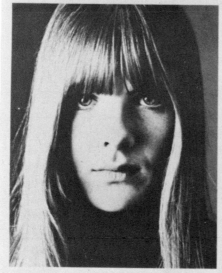

IF YOU'RE OLD ENOUGH TO GET PREGNANT, YOU'RE OLD ENOUGH TO KNOW HOW NOT TO.

We believe that being old enough to have a baby is a tremendous responsibility.

You now have the right to know all there is to know about pregnancy, and the eight methods of contraception.

Here's where you can get this information: Consult your doctor or local health unit or contact the organization below. We'll keep your call confidential.

If you're interested, you're old enough.

FAMILY PLANNING FEDERATION OF CANADA.

96 Eglinton Ave. E., Room 204, Toronto 315

This poster was issued by the Family Planning Federation of Canada. Many of us will use contraceptives only if we are encouraged to do so by imaginative advertising.

method of birth control throughout Latin America.

The incidence of illegal abortion can never be accurately known. Estimates for the United States, before the trend toward liberalization of abortion laws, vary from 200,000 to 1,200,000 a year; for England and Wales, from 20,000 to 100,-000 a year. Because illegal abortion is frequently performed in unsalubrious surroundings, it carries a greater health risk than does legal abortion, and is a cause of avoidable ill health. After the abortion laws of New York State became more permissive, New York City went for six months without one death from illegal abortion. For New York City, that is a fantastic achievement.

Family Planning Is Not Population Control

The ideal size for the human race is a matter of argument. What may be ideal for a conservationist chasing butterflies in the wilderness may not be ideal for the industrialist who wants great masses of people to whom he can sell his products. Since we do not produce enough food to properly feed all of us now alive, many people are becoming convinced that there are already enough of us in the world.

Population size depends upon the birth rate and the death rate. Good preventive medicine and efficient public hygiene have dramatically reduced the death rate all over the world. Most babies now survive to become adults. The average size of family needed to maintain the present human population is one with 2.3 children, and perhaps this figure will soon go down. Since children do not come in .3's, this means that, if we are going to stop our numbers from expanding, most of us can have only two children.

Surveys show that parents in underdeveloped countries want an average of four or five children. In the developed countries, smaller families are preferred. American women in the upper income bracket want an average of 3.2 children, and those in the lower income bracket want an average of 3.6 children.

A useful medical profession can provide accessible contraceptive clinics and abortion on demand, so that no unwanted child has the misfortune to be born. But the medical profession cannot offer population control. Population control is a matter for all of us as a social organization. If we all plan our families to suit our personal wishes, then our population problem will still be terrible. Even if we all became wealthy and opted for the smaller number of children wanted by the wealthy of the world's wealthiest nation, we will, with

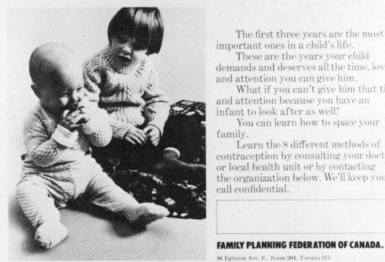

DO YOU WANT TO GIVE EACH CHILD THE TIME HE DESERVES?

The first three years are the most important ones in a child's life.

These are the years your child demands and deserves all the time, love and attention you can give him.

What if you can't give him that time and attention because you have an infant to look after as well?

You can learn how to space your family.

Learn the 8 different methods of contraception by consulting your doctor or local health unit or by contacting the organization below. We'll keep your call confidential.

FAMILY PLANNING FEDERATION OF CANADA.

96 Eglinton Ave. E., Room 204, Toronto 315

Another poster issued by the Family Planning Federation of Canada.

our reproductive enthusiasm, still generate a disastrous growth rate.

There is no simple way to discourage people from having all the children they want. If we replace child allowances with financial penalties, we penalize the already underprivileged. If we pass laws to limit family size, we place ourselves in the invidious position of having to enforce them. If we leave responsible parenthood to the individual conscience, we then select for the disappearance of conscience; and this will certainly stack up disastrous trouble for the future.

Add to these difficulties the perennial opposition of families, nations, races, and creeds to any kind of family limitation, and the outlook for population control is not good. However, without population control, our future will not be comfortable. Like King Midas, who was accursed by his magic wish to turn all he touched to gold, so we—and all those living creatures that are enslaved to our requirements or are dispossessed by our increasing numbers—may live to curse the day when medical science finally gains the power to turn all it touches to life.

SOURCES

Aristotle: *The Politics.* Book 7.

Berelson, Bernard: "Beyond Family Planning." *Science,* **163** 533 (1969).

Blake, Judith: "Population Policy for Americans: Is the Government Being Misled?" *Science,* **164** 522 (1969).

Bose, Nirman Kumar: "Calcutta, a Premature Metropolis." *Scientific American,* **213** (3) 91 (1956).

British Medical Journal: "Ethics and Abortion." **2** 3 (1968).

Council of the Royal College of Obstetricians & Gynecologists: "Legalized Abortion." *British Medical Journal,* 1 850 (1966).

Davis, Kingsley: "Population Policy." *Science,* **158** 730 (1967).

Department of Health and Social Security: *Annual Report for the Year 1969.* London: Her Majesty's Stationery Office, 1970.

Duncum, Barbara H.: *The Development of Inhalation Anaesthesia.* London: Oxford University Press, 1947.

Ferris, P.: *The Nameless.* London: Hutchinson, 1966.

Finch, B. E., and Green, H.: *Contraception Through the Ages.* Springfield, Illinois: Charles C. Thomas, Publisher, 1963.

Goodhart, C. B.: "Estimation of Illegal Abortion." *Journal of Biosocial Science,* 1 235 (1968).

Government Actuary: Office of Population Censuses and Surveys: *Population Projections 1970–2010.* London: Her Majesty's Stationery Office, 1971.

Graves, Ralph A.: "Fearful Famines of the Past." *National Geographic,* **32** 69 (1917).

Haggard, Howard Wilcox: *Devils, Drugs and Doctors.* New York: Blue Ribbon Books, 1929.

Hardin, Garrett: "The Tragedy of the Commons." *Science,* **162** 1243 (1968).

Hippocrates: *Intercourse and Pregnancy.* Tr. by T. U. H. Ellinger. New York: Henry Schuman, 1952.

Lecky, William E. M.: *History of European Morals from Augustus to Charlemagne.* London: Longman's, Green & Co., 1869.

Leder, Lawrence: *Abortion.* Indianapolis: Bobbs-Merrill, 1966.

Littré, E.: *Hippocrates: Oeuvres Complètes. De la natur de l'enfant.* Vol. 7. Paris: J. B. Baillère, 1851.

Murphy, Arthur L.: *The Story of Medicine.* Toronto: Ryerson Press, 1954.

New York Times: "Ruling Seems to Forestall Albany Abortion Debate." Jan. 23, 1973.

Paddock, William and Paul: *Famine 1975.* Boston: Little Brown & Co., 1967.

Plato: *The Republic.* Book 5. Tr. Allan Bloom. New York: Basic Books Inc., 1968.

Rovinsky, Joseph J.: "Preliminary Experience with a Permissive Abortion Statute." *Obstetrics and Gynecology,* **38** (3) 333 (1971).

Royal College of Obstetricians and Gynaecologists: "The Abortion Act of 1967." *British Medical Journal,* 2 529 (1970).

————— Council: "Legalized Abortion." *British Medical Journal,* 1 850 (1966).

Salisbury, Harrison E.: *The 900 Days: The Siege of Leningrad.* New York: Harper and Row, 1969.

Taylor, Gordon Rathray: *The Doomsday Book.* London: Thomas and Hudson, 1970.

Tietze, Christopher: "Some Facts About Legal Abortion." *In Human Fertility and Population Problems.* Ed. Roy O. Greep. Cambridge: Schenkman Publishing Co. Inc., 1963.

————— and Lewit, Sarah: "Abortion." *Scientific American,* **220** (1) 21 (1969).

The Times (London): "Charge Against Surgeon." July 2, 19, and 20, 1938.

—————: "Undue Pressure." Dec. 12, 1959.

Williams, Glanville: *The Sanctity of Life and the Criminal Law.* New York: Alfred Knopf, Inc., 1957.

Useful Doctoring

Even making the doubtful assumption that we can cope competently with the impending ecological and population crisis, we are still faced with the enormous problem of providing ourselves with a just and useful system of health care.

In the rich countries of the Western world, many people are still poor. Low wages, unemployment, physical and mental illness, personal inadequacies, alcoholism, drug misuse, large underprivileged families, small retirement pensions, and inflation are some of the many reasons for the privilege gap between the rich and the poor. Many people need society's care and support; but providing such care already strains our resources.

Helpers and Helpless

Improved medical technology certainly prevents and ameliorates some crippling diseases, but it also keeps alive many severely handicapped people who require long and expensive medical care. Improved medical techniques and better preventive medicine will allow increasing numbers of us to totter into the helplessness of old age.

It is fast becoming more and more expensive to treat sickness and to provide medical care. Government spending increases inflation; and this inflation certainly adds to the difficulties of the underprivileged members of our society. There is no point in any government providing first-rate health services, if the expense of these services causes so much inflation that the old and the sick cannot afford to eat or to keep warm.

As we have more dependent people in our society, inevitably we accrue more professional helpers. There is a real possibility that this ever enlarging bureaucracy of helpers will become permanently poised in impotent opposition to the entrenched battalions of the helpless. The helpers, with their jobs at stake, will make themselves indispensable. The helpless, blaming their continual helplessness on the obvious inadequacies of their helpers, will remain as they are. Helplessness is the easiest of all games to play. More helpers will be called in to do battle, and the helpless will dig into their trenches still deeper.

Sickness has a strong sentimental appeal. It is relatively easy to obtain money for the treatment needs of the sick. But a position may well be reached where, even in terms of health alone, it is more sensible to devote our resources to the prevention of illness rather than to its treatment.

Shifting from Treatment to Prevention

Air pollution, unsafe roads, and unsanitary housing all cause injury or ill health. Even a 50 percent reduction in urban pollution can reduce illness and death from respiratory diseases by 25 percent and add three to four years to the life expectancy of a newborn baby. In Britain, not only do respiratory diseases rival cardiovascular diseases as the number one cause of death, but respiratory diseases are also the commonest cause of absence from work. The man-hours these diseases waste and the expense of treating them makes these diseases very costly, indeed. It is probably cheaper, and certainly more effective, to spend money treating factory chimneys and automobile exhaust systems than to spend money on trying to recondition pollution-damaged lungs.

The cost of patching up people after road accidents is enormous. It is more economical to spend money on road safety than on hospitals to treat the injured.

Unsanitary houses and slums also cause disease. Money spent on housing would probably do more to promote good health than money spent on treatment. The director of the University of Montreal hospitals suggests that the city would do better to spend its money on getting rid of its rats rather than on providing treatment for the rat bites children suffer while playing at home.

Treating illness and providing help uses up human resources at the expense of other aspects of our lives. Over the past 50 years, the rate of increase of doctors per million of England's population has been 1.25 percent annually. A Government report envisions that the annual rate of doctor increase will continue at 1.3 percent. At this rate, in 500 years everyone in England will be a doctor.

The Purpose of Health

Health is a means, not an end. It is a means to enable people to live full and creative lives. There is little point in keeping people alive in an environment so gray and in a culture so dreary that life itself loses its meaning. An individual who is overly concerned with staying well slips easily into semi-invalidism.

Similarly, a society that concentrates on the narrow concern of health diminishes its vitality. If the interests of society are not to degenerate into hypochrondriacal preoccupations, then society, like any healthy individual, must devote most of its resources to the whole process of living and not just to the needs of sickness. The only possible way we can control the economic cancer of health care is to determine how much of our resources we want to devote to ill health; and having done so, then to decide what treatments we can do without.

Are we going to spend our money on heart transplants for physically indolent, overweight middle-aged smokers—or on proper health care for the young? Are we going to spend our health money on large impersonal hospitals, on hospitals which will probably insist on using their expensive machinery to force life into us even when we are old, unhappy, and worn out? Or will we spend our health money on a more personal and friendly service that will cater to our individual needs? Are we going to spend our health money on large salaries for bright nurses, or on small salaries for stupid ones? Decisions of this sort are of course being made in a haphazard way all the time; but more and more, they are being made by centralized, and often rather hostile, health bureaucracies.

Community Health Centers

Many people interested in health care, myself included, believe the present organization of health services is completely wrong. Health care should be brought back to our own homes, to our own families, to our own neighborhoods, to our own family doctors. Care should be based not on a hospital, but on a community health center where care would be more personal, more effective, and less expensive, and where we could all have a much greater say in the kind of services we want.

The arguments in favor of health-center-based care are strong. Such centers could go a long way toward reducing some of the dreadful problems that now confront all the developed countries of the world.

A community health center must be housed in a building specially designed to accommodate all the medical and social care facilities and staff needed to promote the individual and general good health of the people in its surrounding community. A community health center is particularly concerned with the prevention of disease and injury; and in providing help for the sick and disabled within their own homes. A community health center offers care to all the sick, excepting those who require the 24-hour nursing and medical care that only a hospital can provide.

A number of community health centers would share a back-up hospital to which such sick patients are referred. A community and its center *together* determine the policies of the center, and the nature and extent of the work.

Some experts on health care prefer the term "community care unit" or "health center" to community health center. Those less radical in their approach do not see as comprehensive a role for the community health center as the one that I have described. In these last three chapters, I will explain why health care based on health centers will work better than the present system.

The Three Types of Preventive Medicine

Present health care is weighted in favor of the treatment of disease rather than in its prevention. It would be better for both our health and our pocketbooks if things were the other way round. A health center can redress the balance.

For convenience, medical science classifies the prevention of illness under three headings:

(A) Primary prevention is the prevention of an illness in the first place.

(B) Secondary prevention is the detection of an illness in its earliest stages.

(C) Tertiary prevention consists of all those rehabilitative measures that reduce the debilitating after-effects of a serious illness.

In examining each of these modes of prevention, we will see why the health center is uniquely suited to the demands of preventive medicine.

Primary Prevention

Of the three kinds of prevention, primary prevention is the most useful. Medical science can help determine the causes of disease, but it cannot always remove these causes. Much primary prevention lies beyond the competence of the medical profession. Doctors cannot purify the atmosphere, build safer roads, or build more healthful houses. Nevertheless, as a doctor becomes more concerned with the general health of his particular community, he becomes more interested in and vocal about the removal of the causes of ill health.

Socially conscious doctors would be prepared to make "treatment" less expensive, so that governments, after they had paid for medical services, would have more money left to spend on cleaner air, safer transport, and better housing. Cutting the cost of medical care is perhaps the largest contribution that doctors can make to our good health.

Although there is a great deal of primary prevention that doctors cannot do, the primary prevention they can do remains their most useful contribution to our good health. Public health doctors control the spread of many killing diseases. It is they who help keep typhoid and cholera out of our drinking water. If they did not do this, epidemics of these diseases would kill us by the thousands.

Clinical doctors also provide primary prevention of illness. Maternity, child, and immunization clinics, perhaps more than any other clinical tasks that doctors perform, insure that most of us will survive at least to late middle age.

Some doctors give contraceptive advice. Of all forms of preventive medicine, contraception is now the most important; without it, we cannot for one moment expect our communities to remain healthy.

Cajoling the Patients

To be effective, the clinical procedures for the primary prevention of illness not only have to be available, but these clinical procedures have to be promoted. Without encouragement, people do not use them. Most mothers have to be chased, coaxed, and encouraged into taking their babies to be immunized, or into giving their tots a daily dose of vitamins.

Wayward girls have to be hassled into using contraceptives; pregnant women need to be constantly reminded to take their iron pills.

Montreal, the city which spends its health money on treating rat bites rather than getting rid of the rats, spends a fortune on fancy treatments. Each year, the hospitals of Montreal admit more than 250 children suffering from the effects of vitamin D deficiency, a condition easily prevented by providing children with cod liver oil or any other source of vitamin D. Montreal has some of the best and most expensively equipped hospitals in the world; but the city's medical services program would be more useful if some of the illnesses were prevented in the first place.

English children are provided by their government with cod liver oil; but only about 8 percent of the cod liver oil to which children are entitled is actually dispensed by public health clinics. The richest and the poorest cannot be bothered to visit these public health clinics; and it is, of course, the poor who are most susceptible to dietary deficiency. Nutritionally deprived children have an inauspicious start in life, one of the reasons why poor children stay poor.

The Advantages of the Health Center

A health center is just about the best place on which to base the clinical procedures of primary prevention. In this regard, a health center is better than a hospital because it is more accessible. A health center is better than a private doctor's office because the health center has a clerical staff, and also has a staff of home visitors who can chase after the forgetful members of the community. Doctors, in fact, need do very little of the routine work of clinical primary prevention. That work can be adequately performed by competent nurses and a clerical staff. This arrangement, needless to say, economizes on expensive doctor time.

Good health can often be learned; a learning program is a useful part of staying well. Smoking is a health hazard. If we all stopped smoking, there would be less illness in the community. A cessation of smoking could add, on the average, several years to our lives. Doctors know the facts about cigarettes, and as a group, have significantly reduced their smoking. But doctors have not managed to teach their patients the dangers of smoking. Certainly, they have launched campaigns to advertise the danger of cigarettes. Those campaigns have made people anxious, but have not stopped people from smoking. The health center is the place where experiments can be made to discover more effective ways of teaching good health habits.

As families become smaller, young parents know less about small children; often these parents have not seen younger brothers and sisters cared for and fed. Such parents seek information on all sorts of health subjects. The health center can provide this information through films and discussion groups. We do not always need to be looked after by health professionals; given the opportunity, we can often learn to look after ourselves.

Achieving the scientific miracle of organ transplant is fun for doctors. Undoubtedly, such fun is the spice of life. But such medical miracles do little toward keeping most of us healthy. It is the simpler and rather arduous tasks of preventing disease and promoting a healthy life style that are so all important.

The Chinese Model

China is reported to have halved the usual six years of medical training. The government has banned all medical journals. Doctors undistractedly concentrate on preventive medicine, on contraception, and on information about the spread of infectious diseases. Doctors also train peasants, housewives, and factory workers to be paramedics or "barefoot doctors," who then, within their small areas of jurisdiction, keep records on such things as immunization and the contraceptive methods used by women.

Whatever the virtues of acupuncture may be, the Chinese have not lagged behind the West in the oddity of their treatment enthusiasms. It is particularly characteristic of Chinese medicine to have held the healing properties of dragon bones in high regard, and because of this the Chinese have consumed large quantities of fossil bones. It has been suggested that the priceless 500,000-year-old bones of the famous Peking man, which disappeared during the Japanese invasion, were by misadventure swallowed for medicinal purposes.

Still, by concentrating on preventive medicine, China has revolutionized its health care, and China's good health is said to be increasing by leaps and bounds. In the West, it is the cost of medical care that does so.

Secondary Prevention

Secondary prevention is the detection of illness in its earliest stages. If you have a serious physical illness, your chances of being cured are usually better if that illness is discovered early. This observation may not apply to mental illness; studies suggest that many conventional psychiatric treatments only make their recipients more sick.

Mass X-ray, through its widespread detection of tuberculosis, has made it possible to almost eradicate tuberculosis from our communities. Many mass-screening techniques are still in the experimental stage, but some of them will, in time, become important health measures. The health center is the best place in which to organize these techniques.

Tertiary Prevention

The tertiary prevention of disease consists of all those rehabilitative measures that reduce the debilitating after-effects of a serious illness. A serious sickness, mental or physical, is accompanied by the disruption of the patient's life. Often, such a patient becomes physically, emotionally, and financially dependent upon others. On recovery from such an illness, many people need help in adjusting themselves again to the demands of an independent life.

The kind of help needed is varied: a man with a stroke needs physiotherapy to help him use his remaining muscle power to its greatest advantage. A man with a head injury requires retraining in a sheltered workshop before he can hold down a job again in the open market. A housewife who is recovering from a long illness needs practice in cooking and shopping before she can look after her family again. A man convalescing from a coronary thrombosis is sometimes helped if he is progressively given more vigorous exercises.

By using an initial period of gentle training, one Canadian

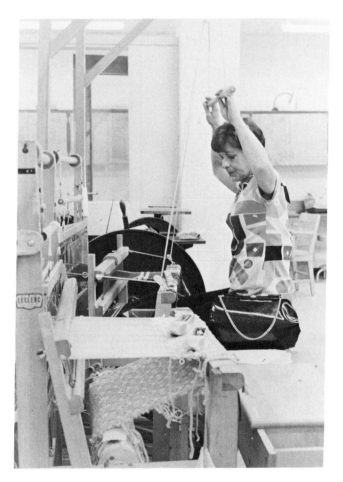

Rehabilitative measures reduce the debilitating mental and physical after-effects of a serious illness. A community health center enables a patient to leave the hospital bed and use health services when he needs them.

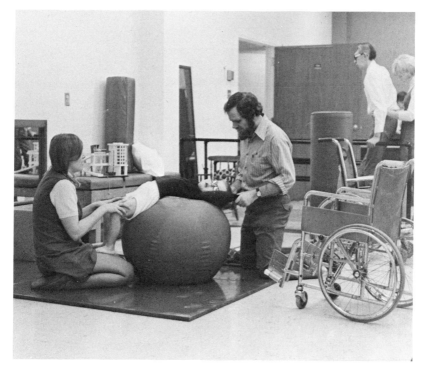

Post-operative exercises in a health center.

rehabilitation center now has some post-coronary patients running a mile in 8.5 minutes or less. This makes it less likely that any of these patients will get another coronary; it also stops them from regarding themselves as invalids. As one leading heart specialist has said: "People need to get off their pills and onto their legs."

At present, most rehabilitation services, when they are provided at all, are provided in a hospital. This means that a convalescent patient must either stay in the hospital to use these services, or if he is discharged, he will go without them. When rehabilitation services are located in a health center, the convalescent patient can make use of them when needed

—which means when he no longer needs the 24-hour nursing and the medical care that a hospital provides.

A lack of hostels, halfway houses, and boarding homes—and a lack of any effective organization in the community to supervise the use of such facilities even when they exist—means that many mentally sick and handicapped patients are kept in a hospital simply because there is nowhere else for them to go. One study of patients in the English hospitals for the mentally sub-normal indicated that only about half of these patients required the kind of care afforded only in a hospital.

A hospital often has a disastrous effect on the mentally ill. Because of this fact, many mental hospitals are trying to reduce the stay of their patients to a minimum. One mental hospital in Connecticut, by the efficient use of community services, now discharges 80 percent of its admissions within three days. Many mental hospitals would like to follow this example, but often their patients, having no homes or families, have nowhere besides the hospital to stay.

What a Health Center Can Do

A health center can run a hostel, a day-treatment center, a re-training workshop, a department of occupational therapy, a department of physiotherapy, and other rehabilitation services. A health center also helps the chronically sick and the disabled to stay at home, and not go to a hospital. As prevention advances, acute illnesses become less common. Many infectious diseases are now prevented altogether; others are quickly cured by antibiotics without the need for hospitalization.

Because people now live longer, the diseases of old age are becoming more common; once acquired, these degenerative illnesses last for the rest of life. The acute diseases once kept doctors on a spritely hop; but now chronic diseases provide today's physicians with a more unleavened load of daily work. Diseases like osteoarthritis, chronic schizophrenia, and arteriosclerosis are the problems of modern medicine.

The needs of the acutely ill and the chronically ill differ. The acutely ill need rest; the chronically ill need activity. A child with acute rheumatic fever or a woman with pneumonia should stay in bed. A man with acute schizophrenia probably needs the protective environment of a hospital ward. But if a woman with osteoarthritis is put to bed, she just stiffens up; and if a man with chronic schizophrenia is kept in a hospital he loses all his social skills. The chronically sick for whom rest is prescribed often remain at rest for the remainder of their lives. Whether their handicap is mental or physical, the most satisfactory way for the chronically sick to remain active is by continuing to cope with the everyday problems of life.

Help is useful when it helps the handicapped person to deal with those problems he cannot manage by himself; or when such help aids him in learning new skills to replace those he has lost. An old lady who has had a stroke may continue to live happily in her own home if she is given volunteer help with her weekly shopping. A construction worker whose leg has been amputated may become a productive member of society again if he is given training for a sedentary occupation.

A health center is designed to provide care for the sick or disabled people who remain outside a hospital. If such people are to avoid going to a hospital they must, at least in part, be able to help themselves. Therefore a health center, unlike a hospital, remains concerned with what its patients can do—not with what they *cannot* do. In short, a health center can help people stay human.

Is Medical Care a Human Right?

A health center is also useful because it makes it possible to set limits on the amount of help provided to the community and to the individual. Ever since the French Revolution, the "Rights of Man," although they have not always been upheld, have certainly been loudly proclaimed. The "Universal Declaration of Human Rights" of the United Nations declares

"man's right to medical care and necessary social services."
Only Gandhi dissented to this human right.

Most Western countries are now embarked on exciting experiments in social justice, and in making social and medical help more freely available. But these programs are often established with a naiveté that foreshadows their failure. Gandhi was more realistic when he maintained that "man has no rights whatsoever than those earned by his own responsible behavior."

If we insist that it is everybody's *unconditional right* to receive medical and social care, our experiments in health care will probably fail. Such an expectation inevitably overburdens the helping services. Also, it is probably not even helpful for our own well-being to regard help from others as a legitimate right. Such an expectation certainly infringes upon the rights of professional helpers who are often forced to provide care when they do not want to, and upon the rights of the rest of the community who have to pay for such care.

The extent to which society can usefully take responsibility for the treatment and care of its individual members can be determined only by experiments in delivering health care. We are less likely to become polarized into the helpers and the helpless if each one of us is expected to take at least some responsibility for himself. It would, indeed, be a poor life if we could not choose to get drunk on a Saturday night, or even if we could not choose to swallow a handful of pills whenever we are crossed. But if we choose to live recklessly, must somebody else always pick up the pieces? A society that decides to do that must inevitably restrict the rights of an individual to injure himself.

Faced with the enormous cost of trying to rescue teenagers from drug addiction, society now puts pot smokers in jail. Paternalistic care and freedom are not easily compatible. Which do we value most? For the sake of liberty, our good health, and our pocketbooks, there is something to be said for retaining some responsibility for ourselves rather than transferring it all into the hands of professional helpers.

Gathering Help from All Directions

Under the present system of health care, a multiplicity of often competing helping agencies provide social and medical care. This makes it virtually impossible both to organize care so that it is used to best advantage or to set limits to its often unnecessary and useless consumption. When several agencies are responsible for providing care, they often end up by providing duplicate care to the help-demanding members of the community, but no care at all for the more undemanding, whose needs may be very real.

There are innumerable examples of this. The elderly indigent in need of public assistance is shunted from nursing home to hospital and back again to nursing home. The hospital argues that old people are incapacitated because they are old, and that they need only nursing care. The nursing home argues that old age is a sickness, and that the elderly therefore need hospital care. The end result could well be, in any instance, that no one looks after a certain old man. Care is responsible when it comes from only one source; then everybody knows who is providing that care or who is not providing the needed care.

A health center, being totally responsible for providing care to its own particular community, is less likely to leave the incapacitated uncared for. The potential problem of bouncing an unwanted patient from a health center to the ward of its back-up hospital can be solved: make the center pay out of its budget for the care that the back-up hospital provides for that center's patients.

Under this plan, a hospital would be supported by its satellite health centers in direct proportion to the services the hospital provides. Such a cost arrangement would discourage any health center from keeping its unwanted patients in a hospital. Such an arrangement would also make it possible for the center to decide how much of its money is to be spent on hospital treatments and how much of its money on other kinds of medical care.

The Doctor-Patient Relationship in a Health Center

A health center would be run by a policy-making board. On this board, there should sit representatives of its staff, representatives of the community the center serves, and representatives of the funding agency for the center. The funding agency may be federal, or state, or local government, or a combination of any of them. This policy-making board would decide how to deploy the resources of the center to most effectively meet the needs of the community. Such a policy-making board would also be ideally constituted to adjudicate disputes between the providers of health and its consumers.

When a patient must pay a doctor for treatment, the doctor often encourages the patient to seek help for every minor discomfort; in other words, to be as dependent as possible. The high cost of medical attention discourages the patient from visiting the doctor too often. But when a patient does not have to pay for treatment, his repeated visits and his repeated demands often become irksome to his doctor. In turn, the physician's indifference becomes vexatious to the patient. Only too often do both patient and doctor manage to tyrannize each other.

One way out of this unrewarding situation is for the doctor, or any other professional helper, to make an informal contract with the patient. The doctor negotiates with his patient exactly what help he is prepared to give, and what cooperation he expects in return. This bargaining arrangement between doctors and patients is already used in many adolescent units, and in some hospitals which specialize in the treatment of alcoholism. An alcoholic requests help for his drinking problem. The hospital or doctor agrees to help him provided that he does not drink while he is under treatment; if he drinks, he will be discharged. Both patient and doctor know where they stand.

The suggestion that conditions be attached to a patient-doctor relationship may arouse indignation. Doctors are notoriously authoritarian; to allow them to negotiate may seem an augmentation of one of their worst characteristics.

Many people—and indeed many doctors themselves—regard it as the doctor's duty to serve all patients. But only too soon does a servant become indispensable, and then turn into a master. Rather, it is in the interest of both the patient and society to have the doctor, and other helpers as well, state exactly what help they are prepared to give, and what cooperation they expect in return.

When informal treatment contracts are used by professional helpers and their patients, inevitably there are times when a patient regards the care that the helper offers as insufficient or unuseful, or concludes that the terms of his contract are unreasonable. The patient, quite rightly, complains to the helper's employer. If this employer is the government, then the professional helper is practically always found to be in the wrong and the patient to be in the right. Greater demands are always made on public servants than on private servants, and the "suffering patient" has the public's sympathy. When it comes to the crunch, informal treatment contracts are always rescinded; and the patient can continue to behave as waywardly as he pleases with the certainty that his professional helpers will have to continue to help him.

But the policy-making board of a health center can ideally adjudicate between the patient and his helper. The board is concerned not only with the interests of the individuals of the community but also with the efficiency of the center and with the morale of its staff. If an individual is allowed to misuse services, then the center's efficiency is reduced and the community suffers. A local policy-making group is, therefore, much more likely to uphold any sensible informal contract than would a remote government official.

Health Center vs. Hospital

A large hospital is expensive to build, expensive to operate, and expensive to staff. In contrast, a health center, with its smaller back-up hospital, is less costly to build and to run, and easier to staff.

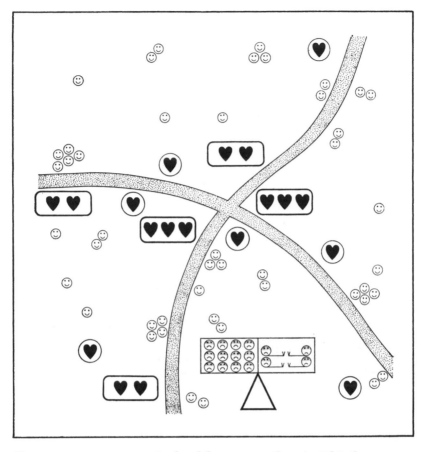

Present arrangements for health care are chaotic. This figure shows a typical town of 100,000 people centered on the crossing of two main roads. General practitioners ☺ work singly or in groups throughout the town. Also working throughout the town are social workers ♥, who are collected together in agencies of various assortments and sizes. The hospital shown in the bottom right-hand corner is overflowing with outpatients ☻ while serving its expensive inpatients ☹ᵧ. The hospital has a supporting industrial complex △ consisting of the laundry, catering service, and central sterilizing service.

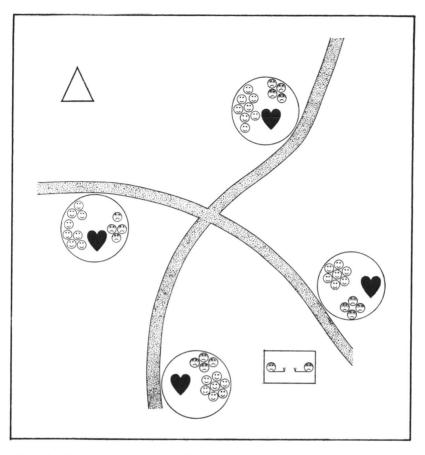

Here health care has been tidied up with health centers.
Doctors and other professional helpers all work together in the
community's health centers. Each center provides all the
medical and social care services for its surrounding community.
The hospital is now smaller, and the number of its expensive
beds is reduced. Hospital specialists see patients in the health
centers, thus eliminating the overcrowded outpatient depart-
ment. And finally, the hospital's supporting services complex
has been moved to the industrial part of town, where it can
serve both the health centers and the hospital. This diagram and
the one on the facing page are adapted from diagrams in
Peter Draper's "Community Care Units: What Should Be Done,"
Medical World, *Vol. 107 (3) 1969.*

Health care is a service industry that employs large numbers of expensively trained staff, mostly women and mostly married. Homemaking women do not like long, time-consuming journeys to work. Many married nurses, social workers, and women doctors lead only partially rewarding domestic lives. The prospects of a job in a far-away hospital may not bring those women into the labor market. The female employee of a health center may have only a short bus ride down the road to get to work.

Where a family's problems are too complex, too many helpers become involved. Such a situation is better managed by a health center. The health center is likely to be more nimble-witted in its responses. A health center unites all professional helpers in one organization, and the center is responsible for the help provided. The help any family is being given is known and measurable. Because the center is the only source of help, it can insist on some cooperation in return for its help. This does, at least, give the family a sporting chance to recover.

Acting as the outpatient department of a hospital, the health center would be equipped with X-ray and other diagnostic facilities necessary for routine clinical investigations. Regular visits by specialists from its supporting hospital would supplement the general staff.

Bridging the Gap Between G.P. and Specialist

This arrangement offers several advantages. Being able to see a specialist at a health center may save a long journey to a hospital. The arrangement also avoids the anonymous indignity of an overcrowded outpatient department. In England, only about one-fifth of the patients seen in a hospital outpatient department are subsequently admitted to the hospital. About 38 percent of these patients are sent straight back to their local doctors, without even having an X-ray taken and without even having been given a laboratory test.

The general practitioner who wants a specialist's advice

can readily meet with both patient and specialist at the health center. Such consultations keep the specialists familiar with the health problems of a community. But most important of all, the general practitioner remains in charge of the care of his patient. Continuity of care is thus an established reality.

The health center provides the help that family doctors need to do their work. Already too many doctors do not want to be family doctors, and prefer to protect themselves from the tiresome demands of patients by going into research, or into administrative medicine, or into a specialty. Surgeons chop away at anesthetized patients, radiologists sit in darkened silence in their viewing rooms, and pathologists get their patients dead. In many medical specialties, the importunities of patients need hardly be heeded.

Family doctors, however, have no such protection. They must listen to anybody who has a complaint. By insisting on continuity of care, the health center makes it much more difficult for a family doctor to palm off his unwanted patients onto others. They also provide him with support, for without this we are not likely to have any family doctors.

SOURCES

American Medical Association: "Medical News: Montreal Reports High Rickets Rates." *Journal of the American Medical Association,* **207** (17) 1269 (1969).

Bruggen, Peter: "The Reason for Admission as the Focus of Work." Association for the Study of Adolescence: Proceedings of the 6th Annual Conference (1971).

Commission d'Enquête sur la Santé et le Bien-Etre Social: *La Santé.* Government of Quebec, 1970.

Commission to Study the Organization of Peace: 18th Report: *The United Nations and Human Rights.* New York: Oceana Publications, 1968.

Department of Health and Social Security: *On the State of Public Health. Report of Chief Medical Officer of Health for the Year 1969.* London: Her Majesty's Stationery Office, 1970.

Doll, R., and Hill, Sir A. B.: "Mortality in Relation to Smoking: Ten Year Observation of British Doctors." *British Medical Journal,* **2** 1460 (1964).

Draper, Peter: "Community Care Units. What Should Be Done?" *Medical World,* **107** (3) 4 (1969).

———— and Israel, S.: "Community Care Units: Staffing and Economic Aspects." *Journal of the Royal College of Physicians,* **2** 251 (1968).

Forsyth, G., and Logan, R.: *Gateway or Dividing Line? A Study of Hospital Outpatients in the 1960's.* London: Oxford University Press, 1968.

Golombek, Harry: "The Therapeutic Contract with Adolescents." *Journal of the Canadian Psychiatric Association,* **14** 497 (1969).

Kavanagh, T., Shephard, R. J., and Doney, H.: "Exercise and Hypnotherapy in the Rehabilitation of the Coronary Patient." *Archives of Physical Medicine and Rehabilitation,* **51** 578 (1970).

Korcok, Milan: "Quebec Faces Health Care Shakeup." *Medical Post,* **7** (19) 1 (1971).

Lave, Lester B., and Seskin, Eugene P.: "Air Pollution and Human Health." *Science,* **169** 723 (1970).

McKeown, T., and Leck, L.: "Institutional Care of the Mental Subnormal." *British Medical Journal*, 3 373 (1967).

Ministry of Health: *Annual Report for the Year 1960*. London: Her Majesty's Stationery Office, 1961.

————: *Report of the Joint Committee on Welfare Foods*. London: Her Majesty's Stationery Office, 1957.

Naughton, J., Bruhn, J. G., and Lategola, M. T.: "Effects of Physical Training on Physiologic and Behavioral Characteristics of Cardiac Patients." *Archives of Physical Medicine and Rehabilitation*, 49 131 (1968).

Office of Health Economics: *Building for Health*. London: 1970.

————: *Malnutrition in the 1960's?* London: 1967.

Owen, David, Spain, B., and Weaver, N.: *A Unified Health Service*. London: Pergamon Press, 1968.

Royal Commission on Medical Education, 1965–68: *Report*. London: Her Majesty's Stationery Office, 1968.

St. John-Brooks, W. H.: "A Measure of Sliding Sand." *British Medical Journal*, 3 407 (1969).

Standing Medical Advisory Committee. *The Organization of Group Practice*. London: Her Majesty's Stationery Office, 1971.

Tendulka, D. G.: *Mahatma. The Life of Mohandos Karamchand Gandhi*. Ministry of Information and Broadcasting, Government of India, 1960–63.

Thompson, W.: "Health Centre Care in Scotland." *Hospital*, 65 (1) 11 (1969).

Time magazine: "The Prescriptions of Chairman Mao" (Canadian Edition). Jan. 10, 1972.

Time-Life Books: *The First Man*. In the series The Emergence of Man. Time Inc., 1973.

Weisman G., Feirstein, A., and Thomas, C.: "Three Day Hospitalization: A Model of Intensive Intervention." *Archives of General Psychiatry*, 21 620 (1969).

Wofinden, R. C.: "Health Centres and the General Medical Practitioner." *British Medical Journal*, 2 265 (1967).

———— "Health Centers: Problems and Possibilities." *Community*

Medicine, **126** 175 (1971).

Zelmer, A. E.: "Fear-Arousing Communications in Health Education." *Health Education,* **9** (3) 1 (1970).

A Useful Approach to Medical Problems

In addition to doctors, all sorts of professional helpers now provide medical and social care. Many a person who goes to his family doctor does not have a medical problem. He may have a bad-tempered wife, or he does not like his house, or he is lonely, or he needs a medical certificate of some sort. Or he may have a cold. Such persons do not really need a doctor at all. Other professional helpers can perfectly well take care of them, often with better grace and more skill.

A health center is planned to utilize teams of helpers: there, the work of health care can be shared between doctors, nurses, social workers, and other members of the center's staff. Health resources being as limited as they are, each health task must be done by the least highly trained staff member competent to do it. It is time to stop wasting our human resources and exhausting our doctors.

To be useful, a doctor must spend time in learning something about his patient, as well as in trying to understand what is physically wrong with him. "It is more important to know what sort of patient has a disease, than what sort of a disease a patient has," wrote the great Dr. Osler. There is little point in X-raying a patient's neck when it's his mother-in-law and not his spine that gives him pain. Nor is it useful for a doctor to prescribe expensive, and perhaps dangerous, pills to a woman for her headaches, when she had these headaches only to gain sympathy from an uncaring husband.

Dr. Lonelyhearts

Proper diagnoses and proper treatment usually require that

303

the doctor know something about the problems that confront
his patients; but need a doctor be expected to become emotionally responsible for his patients? It is one thing for a doctor to know that a patient is sick because he is defeated by
his mother-in-law or because she is unhappily married, and
quite another to expect the doctor to do something about that.

Not only is tear-wiping and comfort-supplying hard work,
but it is indeed seldom possible for one person to solve another's problem for him, to give him peace of mind, or to make
him happy.

Most of us seek love and comfort from others. Doctors,
along with the practitioners of the other oldest profession, are
often regarded as a convenient source of such solicitude. This
has probably always been so. Love is popularly regarded as
a cure for our psychological ills; and now that doctors are
supposed to cure all ills, they are also supposed to be particularly loving. This puts them in a difficult spot.

Doctors are probably less successful in providing love
than are their disreputable sisters. This is not because doctors
are particularly unloving, but because they, like other human
beings, are so constructed that they can feel affection for only
a limited number of people; and doctors often have many
hundreds of patients.

Undoubtedly, doctors often collude with their popular
image of the all-loving person, and doctors of the "love con-
quers all" school are two a penny. But the heart of a physician
is seldom as big as his protestations.

When unhappy people actually go to a doctor for love
and comfort, the doctor can usually manage only a professional gesture. He prescribes pills, or if his patient is unhappy
enough, the doctor locks him up in a mental hospital to prevent his suicide. Aware of his failure to deliver love, many a
doctor gets trapped in a feeling of culpability for his short-
comings. He atones by endlessly listening to his patients' sor-
rows, and by so doing turns himself into a trash can for troubles.

Are such doctors really being useful? By prescribing pills

to the unhappy, they turn them into addicts. By locking up the unhappy in mental hospitals, they actually make it more likely that they will kill themselves. By encouraging trouble dumping, doctors not only legitimatize a great deal of socially unconstructive behavior; they also manage to leave themselves no time to be skilled diagnosticians, experts in medical care, or even adequate psychotherapists.

Perhaps doctors should stop trying to be so all-loving. But who then will guide us when we are in trouble? Who will be friendly to us when we are lonely? Who will support us when we are weak? Who will comfort us when the world oppresses us? The answer is that we should be doing this for each other.

Mutual Help—the Best Kind

Bill W., a Wall Street analyst, and Robert S., a doctor, both had drinking problems. Between them, they founded Alcoholics Anonymous to provide mutual support for all those alcoholics who want to give up drink. A quarter of a century later, AA was able to claim that 50 percent of its members attain sobriety. Throughout the world, AA has rescued half a million topers from intemperance. AA's success appears even more spectacular when compared to the dismal failures that expensive mental hospitals have in their treatment of alcoholics.

For years, doctors have been struggling to make their fat patients thin. Seldom do they succeed, though in the process they often manage to get them hooked on slimming pills. The obese are extremely clever in the art of diet cheating, and doctors are far to naive to catch them at it.

In 1961, a fat Long Island housewife discovered that fat people are much more effective in helping fat people lose weight than are doctors—other munchers know at once when someone is bluffing about calories. Jean Nidetch made this discovery when the obesity clinic she was attending issued her an ultimatum: "Stick to your diet or leave the clinic."

Ever since she was 10, Jean Nidetch had been trying to

lose weight and had been excusing her failures with words like "glandular" and "metabolic." Threatened with expulsion from the clinic, Mrs. Nidetch collected some fat friends with whom she could follow the clinic's diet. They met weekly to see how they were doing. So started Weight Watchers. Now it has 1.5 million slimmed-down members in countries throughout the world. The overweight are giving each other tons of encouragement; and between them, they are losing tons of surplus fat.

Foundations and institutes for the study and treatment of the ever growing problem of drug addiction are springing up all over the North American continent. Well-financed, these foundations lavish buildings and medical auxiliary staffs that are both highly competent and well motivated. But somehow these foundations only cure a very few of their patients.

In 1958, Chuck Doderich and a handful of other desperate Californian addicts got together to free themselves from the seductive clutches of heroin. They were successful. Synanon, their non-profit organization, now owns residences scattered through the United States in which their 900 members live and work together, to cure themselves of their addiction. *They* do the curing—they are not waiting for doctors to do their curing for them.

The Buck Stops Where?

The doctor-patient relationship, like any other helper-helpee interaction, often turns out to be about the most unhelpful of all human relationships. Problems have their uses. Once it becomes the doctor's responsibility to solve a patient's problems, the patient can comfortably keep these problems—perhaps even cherish them. It is not the patient's fault if his problems do not get solved—it is the doctor's. In my experience as a doctor, often the easiest way to anger a patient is to deny my competence to help. It is not my modesty that makes him angry; it is the fact I have passed the responsibility of doing something about his problems back to him. If he does not solve his problems, it is not my fault but his. At this point, he can no longer continue to live with his problems comfortably.

When it comes to solving the emotional problems of every-day living, such a denial of special competence on the part of the doctor is usually no false modesty. There is no reason why doctors, as a group, should be more competent in dealing with these problems than anyone else. In fact, because a doctor's training is long, grueling, and energy-consuming, his own emotional development is often delayed. He is often less clued in than the average person about useful ways of dealing with emotional problems.

The health center will make it easier for people to organize to help themselves. The doctor or other professional helper who decides not to provide a patient with constant help can, at least, help that patient by introducing him to other patients with similar problems. These patients can then get together and help themselves.

Group Therapy

Group therapy was first used at the beginning of this century when Dr. J. H. Pratt, a Boston physician, held classes of instruction for tubercular patients who could not afford treatment in a sanatorium. Dr. Pratt found that not only did his patients learn to manage their illnesses competently by themselves, but in the group, they also learned to cope with the many emotional problems caused by their illnesses.

Patients with physical diseases such as diabetes, epilepsy, and arthritis can well be treated by health professionals in groups. Besides learning useful information about the management of their illnesses from each other, the group members will provide each other with a great deal of support for the inevitably tiresome routine that managing such an illness requires.

Dr. Pratt coined the term *group psychotherapy* to denote the use of the group "process" in resolving psychological difficulties. Group psychotherapy really got going in the 1930s when the demand for psychotherapy was so great that doctors economized with their time by treating patients in groups.

Not only is group therapy an economical way of providing therapy, but patients are useful to each other. Doctors are traditionally committed to being protective of their patients. Patients are not hampered by such professional nicety; they are therefore likely to be more honest with each other about each other's behavior. The group situation also provides an opportunity for its members to experiment with new and more exciting and constructive ways of behaving toward other people.

Many mutual-help groups have developed outside *any* medical control. Sensitivity groups, T-groups, and encounter groups are being used to defeat the sense of alienation that many people experience when they live in big cities and work in large organizations. Encounter groups are perhaps the fastest-growing social phenomenon in the United States and are now spreading to Europe. In the intimacy of encounter groups the lonely make contact with each other. Even the executives of big business learn how to be human. Joy in other people is a learned emotion.

Viable groups as well as healthy societies are concerned with human potentialities, are concerned with what we can do. Doctors, in contrast, are traditionally concerned with what we *cannot* do. We are social creatures; we often need help and support from others; but seldom do we really need support from doctors. Doctors are both too protective and too expensive.

The health center is the proper place in which to experiment with a much wider use of non-medical professional helpers. The health center is also the place to experiment with patients themselves in the management and treatment of everyday problems of illness, dependency, and living. Not only is such a course likely to prove more effective and less expensive than our present ways of dealing with such problems, but such a course will also remove much of the oppressive load of patient care from the backs of our family doctors. Then more doctors may want to become family doctors again.

General Practice and the Academy

The general practitioner usually does not engage in academic research. Most general practitioners work in their own small offices. They have neither the time, the space, nor the help necessary to organize research, either into the services they are providing or into the effectiveness of the treatments they use. But we live in a changing world; new cures and techniques are constantly being evolved. General practitioners, who should be learning these new ways, remain prisoners of their own limited experience.

With an open organization, plenty of space, and adequate staff, a health center can include teaching and research for doctors. A university might attach itself to a health center as easily as it can to a hospital.

Until such a union between general practice and academic medicine is made, it is unlikely that general practitioners will ever really know what their treatments actually do and why they are prescribing them. General practice will remain a dangerous mixture of 20th-century science and of medieval witchcraft, not a healthy mixture from which to fashion the body of today's medical care.

SOURCES

Casriel, Daniel: *So Fair a House: The Story of Synanon.* Englewood Cliffs, N. J.: Prentice Hall, Inc., 1963.

Eimerl, T. S., and Pearson, R. J. C.: "Working Time in General Practice. *British Medical Journal,* 2 1549 (1966).

Endore, Guy: *Synanon.* New York: Doubleday & Co., 1968.

Haggerty, Robert J.: "The University and Primary Medical Care." *New England Journal of Medicine,* 281 416 (1969).

Nidetch, Jean: *The Story of Weight Watchers.* New York: World Publishing Co., Inc., 1970.

Rogers, Carl: "Interpersonal Relationships: Year 2000." *Journal of Applied Behavior Science,* 4 265 (1968).

Shutz, William C.: *Joy: Expanding Human Awareness.* New York: Grove Press Inc., 1967.

Wolf, Alexander: "Group Psychotherapy." In *Comprehensive Textbook of Psychiatry.* Ed. A. M. Freedman and H. I. Kaplan. Baltimore: Williams and Wilkins Co., 1967.

Present-Day Health Centers

Health-center-based care is the most logical and effective way of providing a community with medical and social care. Such centers now exist in Britain, in the United States, in Canada, and in some European countries.

Health Centers in Britain

In Britain, the concept of health-center-based care is now 50 years old. In 1920, a Ministry of Health report recommended that personal health services be provided by health centers which would offer preventive as well as treatment services. Nothing came of this report.

In 1944, the government in its White Paper "A National Health Service" accepted the health center as a necessary feature of its proposed health services. The report emphasized that only by working in modern purpose-built premises, and by becoming responsible for *preventive* as well as treatment care, could the general practitioner be linked to a fully effective health service.

The National Health Service Act of 1946 then laid a duty upon every local authority to provide, equip, and maintain a health center. It was proposed that the general practitioners of the community work in this center. The local authorities were to gather in one place all the many services in that community concerned with health.

The stipulations of the National Health Service Act were excellent, but there were two snags. First, the general practitioners were against establishing such centers. Fearful of the

311

loss of their autonomy, the G.P.'s were reluctant to exchange their private premises for those in a center under the jurisdiction of a local authority. The doctors simply stayed in their private premises.

Secondly, the local authorities never liked spending money; they were doubly reluctant to spend it on a health center when it seemed so unlikely that the doctors of the community could ever be persuaded to move into it. During the first 18 years of the National Health Service, only 28 health centers were built in England.

But times change. For good or bad, the general practitioners of England have become inured to bureaucratic control. Moreover, for the doctor, general practice has lost much of its reward. In 1972, 300 health centers were in operation in England and Wales. Eight percent of the general practitioners provided care for 8.7 percent of the population.

This progress in the idea of the health center sounds much more substantial than it really is because the centers in Britain have been conceived and designed with a breadth of imagination that would hardly do credit to a donkey. All of them are far too small to anywhere near fulfill the extensive tasks of the comprehensive health center I have described.

Old Ideas Die Hard

The original health center of the Peckham Experiment with its swimming pool, gymnasium, and rehabilitation facilities, and with its emphasis on positive health, prevention, and research into the health needs of its community, make even the best of the new health centers seem drab and dreary.

Many of the new British centers are, in fact, nothing more than glorified professional buildings, offices for groups of general practitioners. Within one year of its opening, every one of these centers has proved to be too small. Only a handful of these institutions have provision for outpatient clinics. Most of these clinics snuggle protectively within the grounds of a large hospital. One expert on health care has described these new centers as already 50 years out of date.

Other than the innate conservatism of its public and its medical profession, there is no good reason why Britain should not make the changeover from hospital to community-based care.

Britain's hospitals are old, as are most American municipal plants. The average age of the British hospital is 70 years. Three-fourths of these hospitals were built before World War I. Like many an old gentleman from another age, they are unsuited for their tasks. Britain's postwar economy wilted, and the planned replacements did not get built.

Plans are again under way to replace these antiquated hospitals. The authors of an alternative plan to provide community-based health care centers estimate the cost of building the 1,000 health centers with their smaller back-up district hospitals as 2.15 billion dollars. The estimated cost of replacing the old hospitals is 3.36 billion dollars. Obviously better, but old ideas die hard.

Health Centers in the United States

Health care in the United States is much less systematized than it is in England. Because ill health is so profitable, the vested interests do not take kindly to health-center-based community care. Nevertheless, three forms of such care have already been developed: the neighborhood center, the Kaiser Permanente Prepaid Group Practice, and the community mental health clinic that resulted from the Community Mental Health Act.

Neighborhood Centers

Neighborhood centers are the brain child of the United States Office of Economic Opportunity, established in the mid-1960s to try out new ideas to combat poverty. Government-funded, these centers provide comprehensive family-oriented health services to poor communities. They emphasize those services which help people stay well. They collaborate with other programs attempting to solve the problems that keep people poor and dependent. They are geared to break the cycle of poverty. Neighborhood residents are recruited as health workers, as a means of overcoming the formidable communication barrier that exists between the providers and the consumers of health care.

The Economic Opportunities Act specifies that health services to the poor must be furnished "in a manner most responsible to their needs and with their participation." The OEO guidelines stipulate that the policy-making body of each neighborhood center must include at least a 50 percent representation of people who are eligible to receive these community-based health services.

By 1966, the OEO had established eight experimental centers. In 1970, 49 centers were providing comprehensive health care to a million persons.

Neighborhood centers have had their troubles, particularly in trying to satisfy the demands of some communities. But Dr. Bryand of the OEO reports:

> *If the professionals can continue the dialogue, they generally discover that the consumers and providers become more sophisticated, and a better working relationship will evolve.*

In view of the difficult tasks that confront the neighborhood center, it can be said to be as much of a sucess as Medicare and Medicaid have proven to be failures. Some advocates of the neighborhood center are now calling for funds for 600 to 800 centers to serve the 25 million Americans officially declared poor.

Kaiser Permanente

The Kaiser Permanente Prepaid Group Practice originated in Southern California during the Depression of the 1930s. It has steadily expanded; it now caters to more than 2 million subscribers in outpatient centers, clinics, and hospitals in California, Colorado, Hawaii, Ohio, Oregon, and Washington.

Although this group practice does not offer care to a total community, it does offer comprehensive care to a community of subscribers. In each area, the medical resources of Kaiser Permanente are organized into autonomous partnerships. Its doctors are not paid on the usual fee-for-services basis. Instead, all the money derived from subscriptions of membership is handed over to the group's hospitals, clinics, and doctors responsible for providing its members with care. This set-up reverses the usual economics of medicine. The doctors are better off if their patients stay well; the hospitals are better off if they stay empty.

Kaiser Permanente wants its subscribers to stay well. It has a strong incentive to provide them with preventive care, and to diagnose an illness in its earliest stage. Kaiser Permanente now leads the world in developing techniques for making such early diagnosis possible.

Spending money on the prevention of disease rather than on its treatment is an economy. Although Kaiser Permanente is able to provide its 2,000 physicians and 13,000 non-medical employees with competitive incomes, it need charge its subscribers only about $100 yearly, about two-thirds the cost of comparable care in most parts of the country.

Community-Based Mental Health Centers

Community-based mental health centers are certainly no bold advertisement for community-based care. Community mental health is the latest "therapeutic bandwagon." After President Kennedy's mental health message to Congress, its proponents became even more triumphant. By the middle of 1967, funds had been found for 256 community mental health centers in 48 states. Then federal funds ran low, and politicians lost interest; so available money was sharply curtailed.

The existing community mental health centers come in various sizes and assortments; their directors hold to a variety of therapeutic endeavors. Basically, these centers are designed to offer comprehensive psychiatric care. They provide both inpatient and outpatient care, with particular emphasis on the prevention of mental illness, and on education for mental health.

Many millions of words, some critical and some adulatory, have been written about these centers; but because the results of psychiatry are so tricky to evaluate, it is not really possible to make an honest appraisal of their work. Certainly, they were conceived with an unwarranted degree of optimism. The amount of mental illness in America is colossal. Delinquency, violence, alcoholism, drug addiction, broken homes are all on the increase. The community mental health center was established to stem the rising tide of these social ills, and to prevent yet more people from being pushed into the already overcrowded state mental hospital.

The mental health center has probably had little success with these ubiquitous social ills. But then, there is little evidence that psychiatry can either prevent or cure these wayward forms of behavior. Probably, such behavior can be cured only by the vitality of a society that knows what it wants and where it is going. To discover these cultural goals is well beyond the competence of psychiatrists.

The community mental health center provides a more useful service when it concentrates upon the more menial task of providing hostels, workshops, a retraining center, and social recreation for the more severely mentally handicapped members of the community.

At the time of Kennedy's message to Congress, about 800,000 patients were in state institutions for the mentally ill and retarded; since then, the number of these patients has been reduced by about 20 percent. Certainly much of this reduction is due to more liberal discharge policies. But to the extent that the centers have prevented admissions to the larger institutions and have participated in the rehabilitation of their discharged patients, the mental health centers have provided a useful and humanitarian service.

Health Centers in Quebec

Canada's province of Quebec is perhaps going further than any other area in making the changeover from hospital to community-based care. This change has been master-minded by Claude Castonguay, who headed Quebec's Commission of Inquiry on Health and Social Welfare. This commission made detailed researches into the delivery of health in Quebec and elsewhere. The commission found fault with Quebec's ruinously expensive system of hospitals, its high infant mortality rate, and with its average life expectancy which compares poorly with the other provinces of Canada.

When Castonguay was appointed Minister of Social Affairs for the Province of Quebec, he was put in the rather embarrassing position of an armchair idealist who is suddenly given a chance to make real his perfect plans in a rather imperfect world. Nevertheless, Castonguay is proceeding most stalwartly. Bill 65, which became law in 1971, incorporates his commission's findings.

Bill 65 rationalizes the health services of Quebec. It emphasizes the need for decentralization of control, and gives the consumer a liberal share of influence in deciding what sort of health services he wants. Certainly, the Government still hangs on to the purse strings, but much of governmental power will be vested in the 10 regional health boards of the province.

Today, in Quebec, the community health center forms the basic unit of health care. It is planned that the health center will provide for 80 percent of the health needs of the province. The work of the centers will be done by general practitioners working with inter-disciplinary teams.

Castonguay is an accountant by training. He well understands the finances of medicine. Bill 65 dislodges doctors, especially hospital specialists, from the powerful positions they now hold. Needless to say, many doctors—particularly specialists, who outnumber general practitioners two to one—feel threatened by Castonguay's new health scheme. Many specialists, especially the English-speaking physicians who anticipate trouble due to rising French nationalism, are now leaving the province. Nevertheless, many of Quebec's doctors are slowly accepting the concept of community-based care. They can muster few arguments against it.

In Place of Panaceas

Although most of us are not prepared to believe it, there are no panaceas in medicine. Nor are there panaceas for removing *all* the difficulties of providing ourselves with a just and efficient system of health care.

Providing health care will always be difficult, but the community-based health center will ease some of these difficulties. In a world where organizations become bigger and the decision-making procedures more remote and impersonal, the health care center will help to keep the problems of health care at a more human and manageable level. Health services *can* become more efficient, less expensive, and also more pleasant to use. This would, indeed, be useful medicine.

SOURCES

American Medical Association: "Medical News. Can Community Centers Cure Health Problems of the Poor?" *Journal of the American Medical Association*, **211** (12) 1943 (1970).

British Medical Association, Advisory Panel: *Health Services Financing*. London: British Medical Association, 1970.

Committee on Local Authority and Allied Personal Social Services: *Report*. London: Her Majesty's Stationery Office, 1968.

Curwin, M., and Brookes, B.: "Health Centers: Facts and Figures." *Lancet*, **2** 945 (1969).

Department of Health and Social Security: *Annual Report for the Year 1969*. London: Her Majesty's Stationery Office, 1970.

————: *National Health Service: The Future Structure of the National Health Service*. London: Her Majesty's Stationery Office, 1970.

————: *The Responsibilities of the Consultant Grade*. London: Her Majesty's Stationery Office, 1970.

Dunham, H. Warren: "Community Psychiatry: The Newest Therapeutic Bandwagon." *International Journal of Psychiatry*, **1** (4) 553 (1965).

Garfield, Sidney R.: "The Delivery of Health Care." *Scientific American*, **222** (4) 15 (1970).

House of Commons, Committee on Estimates: *Hospital Building in Great Britain*. London: Her Majesty's Stationery Office, 1970.

Kennedy, John F.: *Mental Illness and Mental Retardation*. Message to Congress. Feb. 5, 1963.

Klein, Donald C.: *Community Dynamics and Mental Health*. New York: John Wiley & Sons, Inc., 1968.

Ministry of Health, Council on Medical and Allied Services: *Report of the Future Provision of Medical and Allied Services*. London: Her Majesty's Stationery Office, 1920.

Ministry of Health: *Hospital Plan for England and Wales*. London: Her Majesty's Stationery Office, 1962.

————: *A National Health Service*. London: Her Majesty's Stationery Office, 1944.

————: *National Health Service: the Administrative Structure of the Medical and Related Services in England and Wales.* London: Her Majesty's Stationery Office, 1968.

Morehead, Mildred A.: "Evaluating Quality of Medical Care in the Neighborhood Health Center Program of the Office of Economic Opportunity." *Medical Care,* 8 (2) 1970.

INDEX

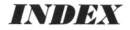

PICTURE CREDITS

PAGE

102   Pfizer, Inc.

112   Dr. Keith Simpson, Guy's Hospital Medical School,
       London.

158   Historical Society of Pennsylvania.

198-   Grove Press Films, Inc., for Frederick Wiseman's film
199   *Titticut Follies.*

216   Metropolitan Library of Toronto.

219   Dorothy P. Rice and Barbara S. Cooper: "National Health
       Expenditures, 1929–71," *Social Security Bulletin,*
       January 1972. U.S. Department of Health, Education
       & Welfare.

233   Eli Lilly & Co., Ltd.

239   Metropolitan Library of Toronto.

252   Dr. Keith Simpson, Guy's Hospital Medical School,
       London.

254   Burt Shavitz.

256   Ministry of Natural Resources, Province of Ontario.

257   British Ceramic Research Association; National Society
       for Clean Air; Pitman's Medical & Scientific Pub-
       lishing Collection—A Regent for the Royal College
       of Physicians, *Air Pollution and Health,* London 1970.

263   American Friends Service Committee.

265   Maurice Chuzeville (The Louvre).

271   Health Education Council of Great Britain.

273   Family Planning Federation of Canada.

275   Family Planning Federation of Canada.

288   Dr. Thomas Kavanagh, Medical Director, Toronto Reha-
       bilitation Centre.

289   Ontario Centre for Crippled Children.